D0384181

From Wellness Experts

"*Mountain Mantras* plays an important role in the movement to improve our nation's wellness. The book is full of actionable items that, if followed, will without question improve one's health—it exemplifies the true nature of wellness, told with a humorous and engaging tone."
— Ryan Picarella, president at Wellness Council of America
(WELCOA)

"Get ready for Kathryn's unique, positive voice. I didn't expect a book about nutrition and wellness, told through the use of a skiing metaphor, to be a can't-put-it-down page-turner. But that's just what *Mountain Mantras* is. Kathryn's personal journey out West provides the perfect backdrop to stories that keep the reader engaged and laughing out loud!"
— Jeanne Nolan, founder of The Organic Gardener and
author of *From the Ground Up, A Food Grower's Education
in Life, Love and the Movement That's Changing the Nation*

"Combining skiing and wellness into a book? The recipe works!"
Juliette Britton, registered dietitian and REAL food
nutrition consultant

"Kathryn Kemp Guylay proves that you can learn new skills and adopt new habits at any age. As someone who's deeply committed to getting people, from kids to seniors, into the kitchen to cook and eat healthfully and be the best they can be, I found *Mountain Mantras* to be a useful, creative, and inspirational book that everyone should read. It offers up a great recipe for success in life and wellness."
— Tanya Steel, Healthy Lunchtime Challenge & Kids' State
Dinner; CEO at Cooking Up Big Dreams; co-author *Real Food
for Healthy Kids*

"*Mountain Mantras* is not your ordinary skiing guide. It's about throwing yourself down the mountain, following your heart, and changing your life."
— Catherine Gund, producer and director of *What's On Your Plate?*

"*Mountain Mantras'* unique approach to health and wellness fuels the mind, body, and spirit. Kathryn Kemp Guylay's experiences, while learning how to ski as an adult, will inspire your greatest potential!"
— Marie Manuchehri, RN, author of *Intuitive Self-Healing*

"There is a wealth of information, inspiration, tools, and techniques waiting for you inside this book. *Mountain Mantras* provides an engaging framework for increased awareness, energy, and overall well-being."
— Sandi Hagel, yoga instructor and acupuncturist, founder of Ebb & Flow Natural Healing

"The wellness movement is gaining more and more strength today, thanks to leaders like Kathryn. I know you will find actionable advice in this book, along with some great belly laughs."
— Elisabeth Grabner, board president of Sun Valley Wellness Festival

"I love how Kathryn approaches wellness from such a positive, nonjudgmental standpoint. You will love her creative games and ideas that will lead you on a path to increased energy and vitality!"
— Kami Miller, health coach, www.mynutritionrenovation.com

"Kathryn has written an amazing book tying together mountains, skiing, and wellness. *Mountain Mantras* gives us a glimpse into her own personal journey out West and inspiration to travel right along with her. This is one book you will not be able to put down!"
— Katherine Sumner, co-founder of Nourish Schools and co-creator of *Super Food Cards*

"Kathryn beautifully weaves together an engaging story to illustrate the interconnection between mind, body, and spirit. Readers looking

to enhance their sense of well-being will benefit greatly from the advice in this book."
—Deb Finch, founder of Deb Finch Healing Arts

"Profundity mixed with home-grown goofiness. Clear, concise, funny, and super-useful. Great insights about key matters in navigating and engaging life."
—Erica Linson, founder of Erica Linson Energy Healing and Classes

"As a devoted advocate for lifestyle as medicine and an ardent, lifelong skier—this book beautifully conjoins two of my passions. There is expert guidance through the bumps here—with wisdom, experience, and humor on abundant display—and the turns, all well carved. Skiers and eaters will find this an empowering, illuminating read."
—Dr. David Katz, co-founder of Yale University Prevention Research Center and author of *Disease Proof*

From Professional Athletes

"Attitudes about nutrition and wellness have the power to drastically alter performance and longevity. Kathryn's lessons are inspirational and practical. All my peers should read this."
—Lyman Currier, U.S. Freeskiing Team, 2014 Olympics, X Games Athlete

"I love the idea of mantras for success in wellness and in life. The lessons from *Mountain Mantras* can be applied to many walks of life, from the Olympics to Main Street America."
—Liz Stephen, two-time Olympian, 2010 and 2014 Olympics

"Good health and a great perspective on life are key elements of success for athletes and CEOs alike. *Mountain Mantras* ties together two of my biggest life pursuits: skiing and wellness/nutrition. Don't miss this hilarious and important tale!"
—David Currier, CEO—SOLU; U.S. Ski Team, 1972 Olympics

"This book is full of life lessons. Kathryn has a great sense of humor! Don't miss out."
—Muffy Ritz, three-time podium finisher, Race Across America; founder of the VAMPS women's Nordic ski program

"Kathryn has been a steadfast and enthusiastic DIVAS participant. We rant and rave about her attitude and efforts and the progress that she's made. We are stoked by the impact the DIVAS Program has had and are full of admiration for all Kathryn does for the community. We all seem to inspire each other. Read this helpful and insightful book!"
—Danielle Carruth & Nicky Elsbree, co-founders of DIVAS (Die Incredible Vimin Alpine Shredders)

"In a world full of complicated advice on nutrition and wellness, *Mountain Mantras* provides a fresh perspective that helps you cut through the clutter and develop a simple and manageable approach to wellness and nutrition. Whether you are an elite athlete or simply trying to get the most out of everyday life (or both), the advice in this book offers great value to any reader."
—Betsy Youngman, two-time Olympian, 1988 and 1992

"*Mountain Mantras* portrays nutrition and wellness in a laugh-out-loud, funny way. Important and fun! Don't miss this book."
—Tiger Shaw, president and CEO, U.S. Ski and Snowboard Association

"As an elite athlete, I know that the way I choose to fuel my body can ensure success or failure. Our bodies are amazing machines that will serve us well if we treat them right. *Mountain Mantras* is a hilarious collection of story telling and great advice from a Chicago girl turned mountain dweller. This is real life, simple advice that won't bore you or require you spend hours prepping meals. These stories will inspire you to make changes and realize your highest dreams."
—Rebecca Rusch, world champion endurance athlete; author of *Rusch To Glory*

From Business Experts

"Real, practical wisdom for all aspects of life—on the slopes, at home, and in the corner office."
—Dave Belin, director of consulting services at RRC Associates

"As an advocate for strong and independent women, I find the messages in *Mountain Mantras* to be very inspiring. A must-read for anyone seeking greater success in life."
—Candace Bahr, managing partner at Bahr Investment Group; co-author of *It's More Than Money—It's Your Life!*

"Great advice for business leaders seeking the most from life."
—Jon Duval, executive director of Ketchum Innovation Center

"*Mountain Mantras* is an easy read for busy people. You will not be disappointed. It is chock full of reminders and great lessons."
—Dr. Tania Neild, chief technology officer at Infograte

"With advice such as 'get some good boots on' (recognizing the importance of foundational education and experience), *Mountain Mantras* is an inspiring read that can change your world for the better."
—Paul Shoemaker, author of *Can't Not Do: The Compelling Social Drive that Changes Our World*

"*Mountain Mantras* takes us on a journey up to the summit, playfully championing us as we learn about how love and wellness can make our descent down the mountain a delightful adventure."
—Dr. Therese Rowley, CEO at Accelerated Alignment and author of *Mapping a New Reality: Discovering Intuitive Intelligence*

"*Mountain Mantras* emphasizes that you are the result of your own actions. If you want to be healthy, live a healthy lifestyle. If you want people to respect you, earn that respect—give back, do something positive, make a difference in someone's life. And don't be afraid to tackle the hard stuff—that's where the you'll find the most rewards."
—Barb Carr, principal at Carr for HR

"Find your center, listen to your gut, and commit. There is great advice to be found in this book."
—Colleen Scopacasa, sales liaison at Ice Mobility

"As a CEO and mom, I found the simple yet powerful lessons in *Mountain Mantras* to be game-changers for my family and me. What a great book!"
—Rebecca Howard, CEO at PayLink Payment Plans

"With advice such as 'throw yourself down the mountain' (to fully engage in your decisions), *Mountain Mantras* is an unforgettable tale with many concepts applicable to the entrepreneur. Laugh and learn your way to success!"
—Leo Pollock, principal at The Compost Plant

"Learning to smile through adversity is one of many great life lessons Kathryn covers. *Mountain Mantras* preaches a positive, health-focused approach toward life that many can benefit from. People who want to focus more on their health and young people starting their careers should read this book."
—Dr. Rick LeFaivre, venture capitalist;
former VP of advanced technology at Apple

From Parenting and Other Experts

"As a mom seeking new ideas for my children and our family, I loved Kathryn's positive advice in *Mountain Mantras*. Tips in the form of games and easy-to-remember rhymes offer a fresh perspective on this genre."
—Laura Carlin, co-author of *The Peaceful Nursery:
Preparing A Home for Your Baby with Feng Shui* and
co-creator of Inspiredeverydayliving.com

"A gem of a book filled with humor and wisdom."
—Scott Kelly, MD, author of *What I Learned from You,
The Lessons of Life Taught to a Doctor by His Patients*

"Kathryn's gift of combining wisdom, humor, and life experience makes this book a must-read for any family. It's never too late to gain insights on how to incorporate health and wellness into parenting. Kathryn makes it easy and entertaining."

—Jenniffer Weigel, Emmy Award–winning reporter; author of *Stay Tuned, I'm Spiritual Dammit* and *This Isn't the Life I Ordered*

"As Kathryn writes in *Mountain Mantras*, we have so much to learn from time spent in nature. Don't miss this great framework outlining what the mountains can teach you about wellness and success in life."

—Deborah Knapp, executive director of Wild Gift

"*Mountain Mantras* provides wonderful advice for wellness and life. I love the idea of weeding the mind for greater clarity and creativity. Read this book and get inspired to make the most of your life!"

—Chrissie Huss, president of Edible by Design

"Heartfelt, hard-won, and hilarious, Kathryn Kemp Guylay's *Mountain Mantras* applies downhill wisdom to life off the slopes. An exhilarating and inspiring read."

—Caroline Weber, author of *Queen of Fashion*

"As a doctor seeing patients who are endlessly confused by nutrition and wellness advice, I really enjoyed Kathryn's description of the 'squirrel effect'. To avoid getting run over and falling into poor health, follow the advice in this book. Get centered, commit, and listen to your body. There are words of wisdom waiting for you inside."

—Valla Djafari, MD, president of Texas Retina Institute

"Kathryn's wellness advice is basic yet enlightening. My favorite tip is to eat a rainbow of fresh fruits and vegetables! Every parent can gain insight from this book."

—Paulette Phlipot, professional food photographer and co-creator and photographer of *Ripe: A Fresh, Colorful Approach to Fruits and Vegetables*

"*Mountain Mantras* utilizes six universal principles that will allow you to be more successful in all walks of your life. Kathryn's words will inspire you to make changes for the better, whether you are a skier or not. Don't miss this book!"

—Annie Burnside, author of *Soul to Soul Parenting*

"Having lived in the Sun Valley area for nearly 20 years, I now have yet another reason to appreciate the slopes. *Mountain Mantras* is a fun and inspiring story. It is chock full of advice that is actionable and impactful."

—Cyndi DuFur, KDPI FM radio show host of *Talk of the Town*

"Kathryn is a national leader for her work to create better health in our nation. In her creative way, she shares an engaging Sun Valley story filled with warmth and humor. Skiing is a wonderful metaphor and vehicle for wellness and being happy and healthy."

—Dr. David Holmes, Head of School Emeritus; executive director of Strategic Initiatives at Community School of Sun Valley, Idaho

Mountain Mantras

Healthy**Solutions**
of Sun Valley

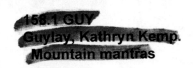
Mountain Mantras

Wellness and Life Lessons
from the Slopes

Kathryn Kemp Guylay

Published by Healthy Solutions of Sun Valley, LLC. Sun Valley, Idaho

This book may be purchased in bulk, with special discounts,
for educational, business, organizational, or promotional use.
For information, please email: kg@healthysolutionsofsv.com

Library of Congress Control Number: 2015911125
ISBN-13: 978-0996532822

Healthy Solutions of Sun Valley, LLC
Making wellness fun.
www.HealthySolutionsofSV.com

Fast and Female U.S.
Supporting, motivating, and inspiring girls to live a healthy lifestyle.
www.FastAndFemale.com/international/usa

Printed in the United States of America

This book is dedicated to
my husband, Jeff.
He has always been there for me,
from bunny hills to
black diamonds.

I love you.

Contents

Acknowledgments

It is with great delight that I take an opportunity to express my gratitude for so many individuals and groups who have helped me on this journey. Writing this book has been like the many other creative processes in my life, based on collaboration and teamwork. Some of you could be named in multiple areas because of how helpful you have been, but I've taken measure to name folks only once. You are just an über-helpful group!

Thank you to my family for supporting me through all that I do: my mom, Marilyn, and my dad, Robert, for showing me that parenting is a lifelong commitment; my sister, Suzanne, for being my childhood companion and setting an academic standard that pushed me to excel at an early age; Grandma Busia for her sage advice and inventive spirit; my aunts, Barb, Candace, Carol, Joan, and Joanne, for setting fantastic examples of how to be creative and inspiring women; my uncles, Bill, Eugene, Joe, John, and Paul, for setting great examples of how to be fun yet dignified men; my stepmom, Judy, and my stepsisters, Joanna and Jessica, for always being so good-natured and supportive. I am grateful for my in-laws, Terry and Wes, for their unwavering support and love. Gratitude for my sister in-law, Sandra, and her husband, Hugh, for being so awe-inspiring. Thank you, Jeff, for always having my back while holding my hand. Huge kisses to my kids, Elena and Alexander, for having unique and special perspectives on the world.

Thank you to my sweet pets for helping keep a smile on my face throughout the long hours of writing: dogs Black Jack and Abby, bunnies Anna and Elsa, and fish Sushi and Wasabi. Thank you to Karsten Fostvedt and everyone at St. Francis Pet Clinic in Ketchum, Idaho for keeping everyone healthy and happy.

For helping to shape the initial idea for this project, I'd like to thank Jane Friedman. For giving me the inspiration to really get rolling on this project, I'd like to thank the folks at Elevate Publishing: Mark Russell, Anna McHargue, Bobby Kuber, and Todd Carman. A huge thank you to the top-notch folks at Quantum Leap for helping me to shape this project into its best form: Steve Harrison, Trish Troilo, Raia King, Martha Bullen, Debra Englander, and Geoffrey Berwind. For their excellent editing advice, I'd like to thank Rachel Shuster, Christina Verigan, and David Yeager. For expert design services, a huge dose of gratitude is due to Laura Duffy and Karen Minster. Thanks to Brad Frazer for your great attention to detail in managing the legal aspects of the project.

My awe and appreciation go to Matt Leidecker for his incredible photography skills and support in providing the cover photo. You are extremely talented in capturing the rare beauty of Sun Valley, Idaho and surrounding areas. Kudos.

A huge thanks to my beta readers who provided feedback on the manuscript, title, subtitle, and cover concept. This book is so much better thanks to your candid and valued feedback: Dave Belin, Barb Carr, Sina Djafari, Jon Duval, Jenny Finck,

C.J. Hughes, Scott Kelly, Robert Kemp, Rick LeFaivre, Erica Linson, John and Jen Neff, Tania and Carter Neild, Holbrook Newman, Rick Shane, and Tim and Corey Zeilman.

More thanks to all those wonderful folks who reviewed parts of the manuscript to check for accuracy and give feedback: Chase Brady, Valla Djafari, Ximena Escobar, Langely McNeal, Leo Pollock, Kikkan Randall, Ryan Redman, Liz Stephen, and Betsy Youngman. A huge thanks to the folks who provided excellent feedback on my cover design, which thankfully brought my team and me back to the drawing board: Wayne Brillhart, Lisa Dirksmeier, Elinor Jannotta, and Jeanne Liston. I greatly appreciate the clarity and assistance you provided.

A huge thanks to my DIVAS coaches for teaching me how to alpine ski, with special thanks to DIVAS co-founders Danielle Carruth and Nicky Elsbree. Your amazing attitudes made this book come to life: Kim Drummond, Heather Flood, Jena Greaser, Erika Hogan, Sonja Huntsman, Claudia Stern, Martina Vala, Hailey Verge, and Davina Walker. You gals shred!

A huge thanks to my VAMPS coaches for teaching me how to Nordic ski. You embody teamwork and collaboration: Kelly Allison, Caroline Droege, Nancy Fiddler, E. J. Harpham, Colleen Hayes, Brooke Hovey, Tess O'Sullivan, Joney Otteson, Susie Quesnel, Joan Scheingraber, Katharine Sheldon, Kris Thoreson, and Kate Whitcomb. Most of all, for her unending inspiration, thanks to Muffy Ritz.

A big shout out to the Sun Valley Company for maintaining the amazing Nordic trails at the Sun Valley Nordic Center as well as Dollar and Baldy mountains. Gratitude to the Blaine County Recreation Department for maintaining the extensive

Nordic trails throughout the valley. We are blessed to carry the title, Nordic Town USA.

Our journey from the big city to a mountain town was made immeasurably more enjoyable thanks to our amazing neighbors, Donna Finegan and Ken Steinauer. Your wonderful horses, goats, and other friends across the street helped make our move so successful. Thank you to Reese for introducing me to the surrounding mountain trails, always with a smile and wagging tail. Thank you also to the Stolley/Drucker family, who bridged the gap between Chicago and Idaho and offered inspiration to connect with nature from gardens to whitewater rivers.

Gratitude and thanks to all of the yoga instructors who worked so patiently over these past 14 years with me as I learned my own practice: Karen Alpert, Kristin Andrews, Mira Binzen, Lauri Bunting, Cara Zaruba Butler, Cathie Caccia, Wendy Dahl, Danielle Fuller, Sandi Hagel, Beverly Hay, Yvette Hubbard, Mac McHugh, Eryn Michaud, Richard Odom, Katherine Pleasants, Barb Sheridan, Jessica Soine, Beth Stuart, and Pilar Tumolo. And thank you to the beautiful studios where I practice and center myself: Gather, Niyama Yoga, North Shore Yoga, The Wood River Community YMCA, and Zenergy at Thunder Springs. I'd also like to thank all of the people who have attended classes with me over the years and shared their energy and practices with me. There are too many to name, but you know who you are. Namaste.

More gratitude for those healers that have taught me the important connection between mind, body, and spirit: Adi Barad, Peggy Bates, Rodney Blount, Deb Finch, Dr. Elizabeth Forbes,

Debbie Garratt, Dr. Jeff Geohas, Julie Johnson, Dr. Maria Maricich, Maria Morris, Molly Peppo-Brown, Dr. Therese Rowley, Sonia Sommers, Irit Steiner, Tif Stewart, Dr. Pieter Van Heule, Annaliese Ware, and Mary Wheeler.

Thank you to the Sun Valley Wellness Festival board and leadership for continuing to bring amazing speakers that inspire me to achieve better health and a better life. The 2015 Sun Valley Wellness Festival, which occurred while I was writing this book, was particularly life changing. Hugs to Elisabeth Grabner, Pirie Grossman, Cheryl Welch Thomas, Dolora Deal, Andria Friesen, Nancy Gilbert, Pam Jonas, Heather LaMonica Deckard, Nick Maricich, Stephanie Reed, and Rob Reeves.

Thank you to the Sun Valley Wellness Festival presenters who were particularly inspiring to me as I wrote this book. Appreciation goes to: Dr. Eban Alexander, Christine Arylo, Laura Carlin, Kris Carr, Kyle Cease, Alan Cohen, Baptist de Pape, Panache Desai, Glennon Doyle Melton, Alison Forbes, Elizabeth Gilbert, Marie Manuchehri, Dr. Sue Morter, Mark Nepo, Karen Newell, Dr. George Pratt, Agapi Stassinopoulos, and Jen Weigel.

I was also writing this book when I attended the 2015 Dent conference in Sun Valley. I was inspired by so many people at the conference, and I appreciated the knock over the head from the universe as the concept of associative fluency appeared again and again. A shout out to Leigh Barer, Steve Broback, Vicky Broback, Cheryl Contee, Sally Gillespie, Morgan Graham, Monica Guzman, Chris Holmes, David Horsey, Scott Jordan, Ann Marie Lipinski, Sarah Milstein, Jo Murray, Craig Newmark, Binta Niambi Brown, Kristen Pederson Galliani, Jason Preston,

David Risher, Therese Tomlinson Magner, Christina Wallace, and Pam Weiss.

Thanks and a big hug to the founding board members of Nurture, who used their hearts and minds to manifest something that is greater than all of us. Juliette Britton, Beth Busch, Cindy Dooley, Stephanie Fine, Julia Goodhouse, Emily Hadley, Dr. Tia Rains, Colleen Scopacasa, and Heather Sullivan. A huge thanks to Lisa Brewer, director emeritus, for her leadership, vision, and amazing ability to write it down. A bow of gratitude to the Nurture Idaho leaders, including Mike Burchmore, Chrissie Huss, Dr. Nancy Mann, Kathleen McCabe, Kami Miller, Jody Moss, Cindi Osborn, Erin Pfaeffle, Paulette Phlipot, Brenda Powell, Janine Seymour, and Julie Siegel. We together salute the Nurture Idaho team that worked the day-to-day growth activities, including Emily Armstrong, Linnea Collins, Madison Hendrix, Missy Russell, Amy Schlatter, Kira Tenney, Stacy Whitman, and Jess Wolcott. A huge thanks to the leadership of Nurture Illinois, with a team including Nora Barquin, Elizabeth Berkeley, Claudia Berman, Alison Bloom, Mini Cheng, Tanja Chevalier, Megan Collins, Allison Farnen, Margaret Frank, Gina Gooden, Kelly Horne, Alma Jasinski, Maxine Manquen, Bonnie Masterman, Elizabeth Matlin, Anne McDonagh, Stacey Patillo, Shana Peters, Eva Pleuhs, Lynn Reiner, Marcela Romero, Kim Seiden, Maize Soto, Kim Treger, Holly Wallace, Brian Weiland, Rebecca Weiland, and Leila Zoghbi. A hug to Matt Hartgering for always keeping our websites in tiptop shape. Special thanks to the many years of service from the Bensman Group and Will Turner's pro-bono legal advice from Barack Ferrazzano.

Gratitude is due to the many teachers and schools that invite Nurture into their classrooms to teach their wonderful kids. We learn so much from working with your students. Appreciation is due to the many non-profit partners, social service agencies, and community centers that collaborate with Nurture to bring the programs to so many people. There are too many partners to list, but I want to offer special thanks to Campus Kitchens of Northwestern University, Family Network of Highland Park (IL), Higher Ground Sun Valley, Northfield Township Food Pantry (Glenview, IL), Presbyterian Church of the Bigwood (Ketchum, ID), St. Philip Church (Glenview, IL), The Hunger Coalition (Bellevue, ID), Winnetka Presbyterian Church (Winnetka, IL), Wow Students (Sun Valley, ID), and the Wood River Community YMCA. I have included a more comprehensive list of non-profit organizations in the Sun Valley community in the resources section link at the end of this book. All of you make this world a better place.

I would also like to thank the large community of supporters that have financially supported Nurture over the years. Your generous spirit and desire to spread health and happiness to the community are truly inspiring. A complete list of donors can be found on the Nurture website (www.nurtureyourfamily.org) under "Give," then "Thank You to Our Supporters" on the green menu bar.

A huge (clean) deep breath of thanks for the amazing folks who worked with our family on a healthy office environment for me to do my best thinking and writing: Dale Bates, Tom Dabney, Steve Kearns, Billy Mann, Thad Nicholai, Victor Vandenburgh, and Gretchen Wagner. You guys are the best!

I would like to thank KDPI FM Ketchum Community Radio for giving me the opportunity to host my own show, providing a great venue for me to meet some amazing people in and out of the valley. A shout out to Laurie Ahern, Scott Carlin, Cyndi DuFur, Dana Dugan, Scott Harris, Christy MacPherson, and Mike Scullion. A huge thanks to my radio guests in 2015 who I have not yet named: Rebecca Brenner, Amy Hager, Trisha Hughes, Brooke Kemmerer, Brad Manuel, Rebecca Rusch, Marianne Ryan, Paul Shoemaker, Katherine Sumner, and Kat Vanden Heuvel.

Thank you to the Community School of Sun Valley for the incredible educational opportunities you have given our family. Thanks also to the Sun Valley Ski Education Foundation for taking our kids under your wings; they have learned to fly down the slopes much faster than both mom and dad.

Finally, thanks to all of the participants in my education seminars over these many years. Teachers always learn so much from their students, just as mentors learn so much from their mentees. Know that your lessons and your mantras are represented in these pages.

Thank you.

Foreword

Are you curious to know what mountains can teach you about life and wellness? The answer is a whole lot! Growing up in Alaska, I have always been drawn to mountains and their beauty. I remember watching my first Winter Olympics at age five. Right then and there, I decided that I was going to be a world-class athlete. Since then, I have competed in four winter Olympics and have been a three-time World Cup Sprint Champion and a 27-time World Cup podium finisher. I was the first woman to earn a world championship medal (2009), the first U.S. woman to podium in the overall World Cup standings (2013), and the first U.S. cross country athlete to win world championship gold (2013). What have all of these accomplishments taught me?

I have learned that success in athletics has so much to do with success in health, and success in health has much to do with success in life. What I love about *Mountain Mantras* is that Kathryn brings together these critical success elements and connects them in a fun, memorable way. She highlights the fact that many of the same skills that make people successful in sports are the same ones that are used by CEOs across America. We all have the opportunity to apply Kathryn's mantras in our lives to excel and be our best.

Mountain Mantras immediately resonated with me. Preserving a positive view (*change your lens on life*) is key; we use positive psychology in many ways on the U.S. Ski Team. Building your foundation (*get some good boots on*) is critical; and as a sprinter, I know that for every minute I'm racing, I'm relying on many months of training. *Zoom out for the best view* is a mantra I personally love, because, even with our training in vision and visualization, athletes can get stuck on what is right in front of them and forget the bigger picture. Setting goals (*plant your poles*) rings true whether you are an athlete, a CEO, or a stay-at-home mom. Remembering that life is long is key. We have the opportunity to achieve so much if we can break down a big vision into smaller, achievable steps along the way. Learning from failure (*embrace the yard sale*) is a mantra that athletes apply regularly. Commitment (*throw yourself down the mountain*) is the most powerful of all. Having the ability to be centered, listen to my gut, and fully engage in what I am doing is a recipe for success that has taken me far in life. Commitment has allowed me to chase my dreams and succeed.

I met Kathryn in Sun Valley in 2015 as part of a tour that included workshops and events for an organization that I lead, Fast and Female. Fast and Female is a not-for-profit organization, started in 2005 by Canadian Olympic gold medalist Chandra Crawford, with the purpose of empowering girls ages 9 to 19 to aspire to sports and a healthy lifestyle. Fast and Female is focused on keeping girls in sports through supportive programming and mentoring from top-level female athletes. Our goal is to provide girls with positive experiences in sports, in the hope that they stay involved throughout their lives. We want these young women to develop self-confidence, a healthy lifestyle, and a positive body image. We also want to demonstrate the benefits of working hard and challenging oneself to achieve goals as both an individual and part of a team.

I hope you are inspired to achieve greater well-being and confidence by reading this book. Keep those mountain mantras in mind as you live your life to the fullest and chase your dreams!

Kikkan Randall

Four-time Olympian and "Get Active"ist
President, Fast and Female USA

ANCHORAGE, ALASKA
2015

Preface

I am excited that you have picked up my book on your journey to greater success in life, whether in your job, at home, or simply through an improved sense of well-being. Are you curious to know what mountains have to teach you about wellness and life? The lessons are many.

In *Mountain Mantras,* I offer up my favorite secret sauces across a diverse set of experiences, ranging from business to parenting to nutrition and wellness. I pull these various topics together through the metaphor of skiing, meant to inspire those that might relate to my own fascination with the grandeur of mountains.

We are all on our journeys in classroom Earth, and we must integrate many factors into the decisions we make on a day-to-day basis. We have many tools at our disposal, including the rational mind, the creative heart, and the primal instincts of our gut. This book is about integrating these resources and applying mountain mantras in order to make better decisions in life.

Mantras are affirmations, highly potent and power-packed formulas, meant to be repeated so you can fully experience their magic. The six mountain mantras in this book are lessons that I discovered through the humbling experience of learning to ski as an adult.

Do you have to be a skier to benefit from this book? Absolutely not. You don't have to live in the mountains or even be in the outdoors to use these mantras to change your life for the better. *Mountain Mantras* is much more than a story about the slopes. It's a Thoreau-like reflection on life and health after leaving the rat race of the city for the woods and the mountains.

In 2011, my family and I made a drastic life change, moving from Chicago to the small town of Sun Valley, Idaho, to get our life back into balance. While I do not expect many readers to be that extreme, I do want you to imagine that you are at the top of a huge mountain, looking down at the many dangers and unknowns that might await you on your descent. Whatever your mountain is—be it a new project, life phase, or simply the start of a new day—visualizing that scene can often conjure up fear and anxiety.

You stand upon that mountaintop many moments of every day. How do you get down safely? This book aims to show you.

As crazy as it might seem, learning how to ski taught me more about success than my decades of professional accomplishments off the mountain. Before moving West, I had been the youngest senior manager in an international consulting firm that worked with Fortune 500 companies; I had founded and grown a successful non-profit organization, Nurture, helping tens of thousands of children and families each year; and I had raised two fantastic kids in partnership with a loving and supportive husband. But I had reached many of my achievements in a frenzied, non-linear, and often exhausting way.

Learning how to ski taught me how to manage the chaos and apply my strengths efficiently. It taught me to see life in a different way. For me, skiing demonstrated that simple mantras could go a long way in restoring order to my life, simplifying the complex, and allowing me to successfully manage fear. I found that repeating these mountain mantras worked well as I struggled to control my trepidation and anxiety while learning to make my way down the slopes. At the same time, I found that these mountain mantras helped me enormously in other challenging areas of my life. Things I thought were impossible became doable. Most of all, I learned not to take myself so seriously!

I am excited to share with you what *Mountain Mantras* taught me. As I spent time in the mountains, for the first time in my entire life, I began to see common themes that helped connect the dots of my various, seemingly unrelated life experiences. Standing at the mountaintop again and again, literally and figuratively, enabled me to put it all together in a way that made sense. What came out of this process of reflection is a six-step plan that will allow you to achieve greater success, happiness, and wellness. These are the six Mountain Mantras:

Mantra #1 Change Your Lens on Life

Learn to look at life in a fresh, more optimistic way, so you amplify the positive elements and filter out some of the negative ones.

Mantra #2 Get Some Good Boots On

Success starts with a strong yet basic foundation. In work and life, securing your foundation can mean putting in time—paying your dues—to gather the experience you need. For example, we teach at Nurture that the foundation of wellness starts with a healthy breakfast and having the tools to quickly prepare simple yet nutritious meals.

Mantra #3 Zoom Out for the Best View

Having perspective on where you want to go and why can have a profound effect on everything you do. We'll practice visualization and manifestation from best practices in the world of sports. We'll also explore how planning ahead for meals can make all the difference in wellness outcomes.

Mantra #4 Plant Your Poles

Having a long-term vision is a great place to start, but breaking it down into manageable, digestible steps is what enables you to actually move forward. I'll share some ways to ensure you stay on track along your journey.

Mantra #5 Embrace the Yard Sale

In skiing, a "yard sale" is an affectionate term for when you fall and lose all your equipment. Skis pop off, poles go flying, and you might end up with snow in every crevice. These failures offer us great opportunities for improvement if we can accept and learn from them.

Mantra #6 Throw Yourself Down the Mountain

Even if you have all the other tools in place—a good attitude, foundation, vision, goals, and a means to learn from failure—you can't learn to succeed until you learn to commit. Following your gut and then being able to commit, based on what your gut is telling you, can be scary. You'll learn techniques for overcoming fear so you can find balance and success in whatever you do.

To be clear, *Mountain Mantras* is not a book about how to ski; it is about how your attitude and approach affect your capabilities and outcomes, with some tips for success on the slopes along the way. Each mantra includes action steps that will provide you with inspiration and ideas for improvement, whether you're a skier or not!

My greatest wish is that you enjoy the journey through this book and your life. I hope that you laugh out loud as you read, even though it will often be at my expense! *Mountain Mantras* is for the life adventurer who is ready for positive change and the reader who welcomes helpful and actionable advice served up with some humor. Enjoy.

Kathryn Kemp Guylay

SUN VALLEY, IDAHO
2015

A NOTE FROM THE AUTHOR:

The stories you will read in *Mountain Mantras* are based on real experiences and real people. Some names and some circumstances have been changed in order to protect the identity of individuals. Some of the stories and quotes in this book have been reproduced from transcripts from my radio show ("Healthy Kids Corner" on KDPI FM Ketchum Community Radio). In these instances, I kept quotations as close to the original as possible. When conversations were not recorded, I reproduced quotes from memory and, in most cases, confirmed their authenticity with the speakers. I reserve literary right to omit or add to these stories to make them more intriguing and make the lessons from the mountains as memorable as possible.

Mountain Mantras

Change Your Lens on Life

**Gratitude, the ability to count your blessings,
is the ultimate way to connect with the heart.**

—BAPTIST DE PAPE
author of The Power of Heart

Viewing life through a new lens doesn't have to mean putting on rose-colored glasses or wishing for a Disney movie ending. Our perspective on life affects how we experience it, how we interact with others, and, ultimately, our wellness and well-being.

Goodbye, Windy City. We're Going West!

I remember looking up at Bald Mountain (nicknamed Baldy by skiers) for the very first time. The mountain embodies winter life and recreation in the beautiful town of Sun Valley, Idaho. I felt its majesty, size, and beauty and thought, "People actually *ski* down that monster of a hill?"

It was the summer of 2011, and our family had just moved out West in a quest to escape the rat race that had become our life in Chicago. I considered myself a recovering management consultant who had survived a successful rise to the top of a great firm. In the process, I had become an expert at memorizing the names of the flight attendants who served my regular routes in and out of Chicago. Yes, I traveled a lot and logged many billable hours on the go.

My husband, Jeff, was an investment banker who had started out on Wall Street before following his career to Chicago. While he loved his work, he had had enough of the stress that drove people to find extreme ways to unwind. One of the most memorable—and bizarre—stories included people running across trading floors and screaming before dunking their heads into vats of guacamole to relax.

We hit our thirties as a career couple and were blessed with two wonderful kids: Elena, born in 2000, and Alexander, in 2003. Parenthood turned our world upside down. We learned quickly that our competitive careers had nothing on the world of suburban baby playgroups.

"Did you get a spot in the baby Spanish class?"

*"I had to sleep outside in line just to
get my little Gracie signed up!"*

*"I feel so much better knowing that my Tommy
has passed swim certification!"*

*"Yes, we got Charlotte passed when
she was only three weeks old!"*

"Which of the 'Baby Mozart' series is your favorite?"
"Peter really enjoys the Rachmaninoff!"

*"In our house we prefer to have professional
musicians play for Cassidy. That way she can
actually feel the vibrations of the music
and fully integrate it into her learning!"*

As Elena and Alexander passed through their toddler years, we tried to keep up—golf pro classes at age two and career coaches at age three—but we were getting tired of the scene. After a few years as both a parent and a principal in my firm, it became clear that a change was in order when we realized that Elena did not understand any English. She was a Spanish speaker, just like her nanny, her primary conversation partner while my husband and I were away working. At first, I thought it could be a great asset and something to brag about at mother-daughter playgroups, but upon further reflection, I opted for a career change. I looked for work I could do from home and secured my certification in nutritional counseling. To get there, I had to earn additional credentials beyond my graduate degree, which took almost five years, not a surprising timeline given that I was balancing part-time work and studying in the few hours a day Alexander was at preschool. While in the homestretch of achieving my certification, I stepped into the non-profit world and founded Nurture, a nutrition and wellness education organization. Nurture is dedicated to improving the nutrition and wellness of children and families, especially low-income families.

I also spent some time at home and spoke a little English with my daughter!

A few years later, we started to vacation out West as a family. We noticed that everything seemed better when we immersed ourselves in nature. Perhaps it was that things were simpler. Jeff had always been a big skier and loved the mountains, while I was a sunshine and water gal. Inevitably, we landed in Sun Valley every year for at least a week or two. I didn't consider myself a skier, but I gave it a try on the bunny hill. It was nothing I was serious about. That is, until we actually decided to *live* in Sun Valley.

The move was a major risk for our careers, but we were willing to take it. By then, Nurture had taken off, and I was ready to hand over operations in Chicago to a new leader while I attempted to expand operations beyond the Windy City. Jeff would travel for his work no matter where we lived, so we figured, with the business world becoming more and more virtual, we could amp up our Skype accounts and head West.

When we arrived in Sun Valley, Elena entered fifth grade and Alexander was in third. They were eager for an adventure and they bubbled over with excitement. We all smiled as we pulled into the mountain town with a total population of less than 1,500. There were only about 20,000 people living in the area that stretched from one end of the remote valley to the other.

Where is everyone?

Is there really only one grocery store?

*Why are there animal heads mounted
in the garage of our rental home?*

Jeff and I had taken a huge financial risk and left behind a wonderful support network of family and friends in Chicago. We knew only a few people in this teeny, tiny town, yet we kept up a positive front and a smile. That was our calling card. Our ability to smile through adversity had been a savior to me, and I knew it was going to save us over and over again as we started anew in this different place.

DON'T BE IN A WORRY STATE.
LOOK FORWARD AND APPRECIATE.

Transform Fear into Love

Despite my professional experiences with demanding clients
and the relentless pursuit of billable-hour targets, what I feared
most in 2011 was Bald Mountain. With Jeff being an accomplished skier, he planned on taking only a few runs here and
there whenever he could break away between meetings and
phone calls. It was obvious that he was not a ski partner who
could help me work on the basics. My kids, then 8 and 10, had
already passed me by and had long since stopped waiting for me
at the bottom of our runs. No one wanted to go on the bunny hill
with me. My kids made rapid progress on the slopes; being so
lightweight and low to the ground made it easier for them to re-
cover from falls. I was taller, weighed more, fell more often, and
quickly began to ache. I developed a hematoma on my outer
thigh from repeatedly falling on it. My neck gaiters (scarf-like
loops of warm fabric) became *thigh gaiters*, as I pulled them
around my legs and butt to cushion my falls. I was getting so
bruised that I had resorted to wearing Jeff's huge and highly
padded hockey pants while I skied. Perhaps that fashion faux
pas was the reason my kids were pretending not to know me. I
needed to find serious ski instruction, and quickly.

I learned about Die Incredible Vimin Alpine Shredders
(DIVAS) from another mom who also was a beginner skier and
had searched for all the help she could get. The Sun Valley
Snowsports School had started this women-only group a year

earlier, and I heard it had filled up pretty fast, so I was surprised to get a spot. "No problem, honey!" said the woman on the other end of the phone line.

No problem?

I had no idea what to expect on our first day of class. "Okay, everyone, we are going up the lift to do a ski-off!" yelled Nick, the red-coated DIVAS program manager. I was a nervous wreck inside. *What did "ski-off" mean?* After snowplowing my way down the smallest hill, I was partnered with a lovely group of grandmothers (cool grandmas, for sure). For the next several months, we skied together every week, talking on the lifts about kids and grandkids. We skied our way down and improved our skills. I soaked up every word that the amazing (and often intimidating) ski instructors offered.

I also did something that transformed my beginner ski status in an important way: I showed up every single week wearing a huge smile. It didn't matter that I often had to alternate these smiles with tears of frustration (whenever my expert husband took me out for a *quick run down the bowls*). It didn't matter that I had to alternate these smiles with looks of shock as I checked out my butt bruises at the end of the day. I simply knew I had to keep smiling. And it paid off.

At the end of my first DIVAS season, I received an honor that made my year: the Best Attitude Award. It made the pain of all those bruises vanish into sweet oblivion. I don't think I'll ever get an award that means as much as that card and t-shirt handed over at a local bar. It filled me with love for my new favorite sport, the mountain on which we played, and all the amazing people I was going to meet.

GIVE THANKS,
EVEN FOR FALLING IN SNOW BANKS.

Embrace Your Inner Superhero

As I learned through my bruising first attempts at skiing down the mountain, when you smile, whether you feel it inside or not, you are sending a signal to your body that *all is well*. When I interview people on my radio show, I always ask them to smile when they talk. Believe me, you can hear it over the air! You sound more approachable and less nervous if you speak through a smile.

Smiling is part of important body language that affects you and those around you, but it's not the only way we can impact how the world perceives us. Dr. Amy Cuddy, who is on the faculty at Harvard Business School and is a researcher of nonverbal behavior, advocates assuming dominant positioning before and during a meeting or talk to give yourself more power and influence. Wonder Woman was onto something when she assumed the wide-legged, proud stance with arms bent and hands on hips! There's evidence that the Wonder Woman pose actually reduces your levels of cortisol (the stress hormone) and raises your level of testosterone (a hormone related to strength).

Putting a smile on your face makes people see you differently. With a smile, you are viewed as more attractive, reliable, relaxed, and sincere. You are rewarding others and yourself when you smile. And because smiling is contagious, others are likely to smile back. By smiling, you release feel-good chemicals in your brain, feel more confident, project a more pleasant voice, and activate reward centers in the brains of those around you. It is always a win-win to smile.

PUT ON A SMILE.
IT NEVER GOES OUT OF STYLE.

When Ants Attack

Back in Chicago, when Alexander was three, we were invited to a birthday party for my dear friend, Julia. We were in charge of bringing a cake and, given that Julia was one of the most accomplished cooks I knew, I felt pressured to find a recipe that would have a wow factor. My friend Chase had recently invited us over for dinner and, for dessert, had served a bundt cake with a delicious chocolate glaze in a beautiful pattern dripping down the sides. Chase had five kids, so I knew she didn't mess around with complicated recipes.

"Just melt some dark chocolate and add a tiny bit of olive oil to give it a smooth texture," Chase said. "Then drip it down the cake in a pretty pattern. It is sure to impress!"

On the day of the party, 30 minutes before we had to leave, I was in the kitchen following Chase's instructions. I had the help and full attention of Alexander as we poured the dark chocolate over the cake.

"Great job, Alexander!" I said, as we finished the glaze. It was just starting to harden, and I did think that it would look beautiful.

"I am just going to go upstairs to take a quick shower before we go to the birthday party," I told Alexander. He nodded solemnly, pretending to go off to the playroom to busy himself.

About 15 minutes later, I came downstairs to find a boy with wide eyes and a huge ring of chocolate around his mouth.

"Mama. The ants. They came. And ate the cake!"

Very seriously, he led me to the kitchen, where the cake stood, yellow and pockmarked. There was not a morsel of chocolate to be found.

"Look, mama. See? The ants!"

I looked at my darling son, with his huge ring of chocolate around his mouth, and remembered the *DO NOT EAT* signs my stepmother used to hang on jars of chocolate chips. As a teenager, I had felt a lot of shame and guilt taking chocolate chips from those containers. I didn't want him to feel that same way.

"The ants did like that cake, didn't they?" I said with a smile. "Let's go wash your face, okay?"

I got on the phone with Julia and gave her the quick story, which elicited huge giggles.

"Okay, I'm good with the half-eaten cake ... Let's go with it." Julia was not only a superb cook, she was also a great sport.

We arrived at Julia's birthday with the cake, and all enjoyed a lovely meal. Our mealtime stories included the mystery of the ant attack on the cake. As the meal progressed, I noticed that Alexander was wobbling in his chair with half-closed eyes. I think he was stuffed full and hitting the sugar low at the same time. I refrained from chuckling, and no one scolded or judged. That day, Alexander learned his own, very personal and memorable lesson about how what you eat translates

into how you feel. Now a tween, Alexander must make his own
decisions about what to eat, based on how the foods actually
make him feel.

AVOID SHAME,
FOR A HEALTHY LONG-TERM GAME.

Transform Unhealthy Relationships into Healthy Ones

I knew early in my consulting career that my positive attitude
would help me get promotions, clients, and success in the business world. This realization occurred well before I read the evidence in Shawn Achor's *The Happiness Advantage.* He found
that performance improvements, such as 37% in sales, 31% in
productivity, and 40% higher likelihood of receiving a promo-
tion, are all linked to happiness. Happy people are nearly ten
times more engaged at work, get better grades, and even live
longer.

I learned the importance of showing up with a smile, no matter how I felt on the inside, from Frank. He was the highly successful head of the Los Angeles office of the management
consulting firm where I worked. I was in the Chicago office, and
it was a rare and special occasion to work with one of the senior
partners from another city. I learned quickly that being assigned to a project with Frank could be a curse or a blessing,
depending on whom you asked. Because of his extremely high
expectations, he was known to work his consultants into the
ground, yet it was also observed that those who worked well
with him moved ahead quickly.

When I was assigned to my first project with Frank, I was responsible for managing my own team of two consultants. Steve and Alice, who at that time made up my small team, had different personalities and would learn different lessons from our project. Steve was new, on the naïve side, and needed guidance. He was the easy one. Alice was extremely bright, experienced, and had lots of ideas. She was the difficult one. Alice often left me exhausted and unhappy.

"Hey, Kathryn! Hey! Do you have two quick seconds to talk?"

"Sure ..."

"Did you get stuck in that horrible traffic jam on 290 this morning? What a nightmare."

"Yes. It did finally get moving though," I said.

"No way. I can't believe how stupid people are. No one in this town can drive in the snow. It reminds me of this time when I was visiting my aunt, who is a terrible, crazy person, by the way, and it snowed in South Carolina. Now THOSE people are *really* crazy!"

"Interesting. I went to Emory and used to visit South Carolina all the time. Loved it. My roommate, a Merit Scholar, was from there."

"Really? I had the worst roommate in college. I remember when ..." Her voice droned on and on and on.

Was she really talking about a toga party in 20-degree weather? Cars breaking down on road-trips? A blind date from hell?

My lifeblood was being sucked by an energy vampire. I looked inward for some positive thoughts, and I resurfaced to the light.

"Great, Alice. I have to run because we need to get busy on Frank's project."

That snapped Alice out of her ridiculous story. She had worked with Frank and knew what lay ahead. The next week was a day-and-night marathon of work as we prepared our client kick-off meeting presentation materials according to Frank's guidance. By the time we reached the client site in California to meet Frank in person, we all were feeling overworked and exhausted.

"Okay, what's the status on the kickoff meeting presentation?" Frank drilled us over breakfast.

"Well," Alice said bravely, "Let me show you on the overview page of our report. I just have to get it out of my bag that hopefully survived the terrible taxi driver that picked us up from the airport. I swear he dropped my bag and had no right to be driving a taxi because he had no sense of direction. And the hard braking was nauseating! Smelled bad in there, too ... I'm sure he had made someone before us puke ..."

"I don't care about your bad taxi driver!" yelled Frank. "And our client *especially* won't care about your bad day, your bad driver, or any bad smell you experienced!"

"Sorry, Frank, it was just that we had a really hard week at the office, and then my cat was sick, and then we had this huge snafu with our contractor that is re-doing our kitchen ..."

"NO talk about your sick cat! NO talk about your botched home projects!" yelled Frank.

People at the Holiday Inn breakfast bar were staring at us. It was an awkward moment but a pivotal one for me. We were professional services providers, and people were buying a relationship with us as much as they were buying a service. Clients expect you to be confident, upbeat, and positive. No one wants to hear about your tough day.

Frank concluded, "No matter what your day has really been like so far, it has been GREAT as far as the client is concerned! Couldn't be better!"

**FOR AN ATTITUDE OF THANKS,
FOLLOW THE RULE OF FRANK'S.**

Food as Fuel

As I later reflected on our breakfast meeting and Alice's trail of misery, I wondered how her days were starting even before she got ready to leave for the office. Now, as executive director of Nurture, with my certification in nutritional counseling, I have gained a lot of experience teaching children and adults about nutrition.

For starters, I have learned that in our American culture, we need to develop a better relationship with food. Eating from fear or guilt is not good for you. Eating to cover up insecure or sad feelings is not good for you, either. If you deny yourself food, that behavior is equally unhealthy. Recognize, instead, the necessity of food as the gas in our tanks and a source of our energy.

We all need to view food as fuel. This lesson was brought home during my 2009 search for a head of children's programming for Nurture.

"Remember that kids have different objectives around food than adults. They want to run fast, feel great, and do better in sports and in school. They could care less about cardiovascular disease," said Juliette Britton, my top candidate.

"You also will completely alienate yourself the minute you say that their favorite cookie or sugary drink is 'bad.' Never use the word 'bad' when talking to kids about nutrition!"

Juliette got the job. I loved her philosophy, and she had the right background. She had been a children's nutrition educator in Colorado and was in Chicago studying to get her registered dietitian degree.

I observed Juliette's teaching style over the next few years, and Nurture adopted her techniques and lesson plans for kids. The key was to avoid confusing nutrition jargon and keep it simple. Lessons start by establishing a vocabulary to talk about food. We call it the *go* vs. *slow-down* lesson, using words that make sense to kids and refer to what they want to do.

Do they care that canned frosting has fats that may be bad for their heart? Not so much. Do they care if eating unhealthy foods will make them slow down, not have sustained energy, or make them sleepy? Yes!

By understanding why the body needs food, it becomes much easier to decipher what types of food provide the best fuel. Any food with calories provides energy for the body. However, not all calories are created equal. A powdered-sugar donut has the same number of calories as a bowl of oatmeal with strawberries and slivered almonds. Yet, while the body feels hungry several hours after eating the donut, the oatmeal is filling and nutritious.

"What foods give the body long-lasting energy?" our Nurture instructors ask an eager group of kindergarteners.

> "Carrots!"
> "Apples!"
> "Meat!"
> "Cheese!"
> "Strawberries!"
> "Broccoli!"

These answers are right on target. Note the absence of low-fat energy bars, fast food, baked chips, and processed foods. The only responses were whole foods, mainly fruits and vegetables, which Nurture calls *go foods* because they fuel the body with long-lasting energy, vitamins, minerals, and nutrients to support growth and activity. *Go* foods include fruits and vegetables, lean proteins, nuts, legumes, eggs, milk, and whole grains. Go foods fuel the body so it can move!

"What foods slow the body down?" we ask the kindergarteners.

> "Cookies!"
> "Cake!"
> "Ice cream!"
> "Brownies!"
> "Potato chips!"
> "French fries!"
> "Candy!"
> "Soda!"

Nurture refers to foods that have little nutritional value as *slow-down* foods or *sleepy* foods. These foods may provide a short burst of energy, but they soon leave the body feeling hungry or tired. *Slow-down* foods slow down the body.

"If *slow-down* foods make us sleepy, does that mean we can never eat them?" we ask the kindergarteners.

"No," they say wisely. "*Slow-down* foods are okay every once in a while."

What I love most about this Nurture lesson is how even kindergarteners understand that *go* foods are the best, but *slow-down* foods can be part of a balanced diet when consumed in moderation. We are not making anything bad or creating shame.

By promoting a positive relationship with food, we are setting the stage for a healthy, energized relationship with food. Energy is a buzzword that is loved by kids and adults because it implies movement and fun. *Go* foods, on the one hand, capture this liveliness. *Slow-down* foods, on the other hand, promote sleepiness. And not many children want to feel sleepy!

**LEARN TO VIEW FOOD AS FUEL,
LIKE NURTURE TEACHES KIDS AT SCHOOL.**

You Are What You Eat and So Much More

I have learned so much from my friends and Nurture board members who graduated from the Institute of Integrative Nutrition (IIN), namely Eila Johnson, Stacey Patillo, Kami Miller, and Jody Moss. These lovely ladies consistently remind me that what we put into our mouths constitutes our *secondary foods*, which are important but less so than our *primary foods*.

Primary foods are relationships, daily activities, and spiritual practices that sustain us at a basic level. These primary foods have a whole lot more impact on our stress levels than what we put on our plates and into our mouths. We can't fix secondary food issues without addressing the primary ones. Ideally, we fix the problems by changing the way we look at both primary and secondary foods simultaneously. Thus, on our quest for better wellness and productivity, adjusting our lens on life through yoga and other practices that unify our mind, body, and spirit, is as integral as changing our views on food and nutrition.

**IT'S NOT JUST THE FOOD ON YOUR PLATE
THAT CAN DEPLETE YOU OR MAKE YOU FEEL GREAT.**

The Power of the Lens

Also from Achor's *The Happiness Advantage* comes the idea of "Falling Up." Falling Up is the concept that failure will inevitably happen, so it should be viewed as a normal, even positive, part of life. Achor believes that people's perceptions are based on their individual "Explanatory Style." Achor advises us to avoid helplessness, a disempowered attitude that generally leads to a destructive path of inaction. Falling Up requires people to look for the opportunity in any setback rather than settling for despair. This proactive attitude is what separates the successful from those who give up.

For me, Explanatory Style is *the lens on life* through which I choose to view a situation. It is a choice that each of us can make every day, many times a day. I like to recall an equation I learned in graduate school that explains how we arrive at satisfaction:

$$Satisfaction = Perceived\ Reality - Expectations$$

What parts of the equation do we control? Both perceived reality *and* expectations. We have the ability to influence our happiness in and satisfaction with life by managing those two components individually.

Let's start by managing our expectations. Common sense will tell you that if you set your expectations too high, you will likely end up disappointed. My advice is that you don't expect the world to be handed to you on a silver platter. Life isn't supposed to be endless leisure and comfort. Life is, in fact, a classroom in which we constantly learn important lessons. Don't expect it to be easy, but don't assume it will be terrible, either.

As you'll learn in Mantra #3 (Zoom Out for the Best View), the law of attraction—the concept that you can manifest things in your life through the power of thought—is an important force. Of course, we have to work hard for our rewards and not just wish for them. You'll learn in Mantra #4 (Plant Your Poles) that I advocate setting realistic, attainable goals as you endeavor to reach your life vision. Along the way, I suggest an even balance between proactivity (working hard) and receptivity (letting things flow to you).

Once we have set our expectations at a realistic level, we turn to the second component: perceived reality. It should be obvious that if you view your reality as poor or low, your satisfaction will also be poor or low regardless of expectations. But why not choose an optimistic Explanatory Style to interpret events? Throw out that pair of negativity-infused goggles and put on some new ones! Make the most of every situation and boost your perceived reality. By looking at reality through a positive lens, we avoid sinking into helplessness and blaming others for our circumstances. Those with a positive Explanatory Style are much more likely to see what they can learn from their circumstances and drive themselves toward higher performance. They are also more likely to be satisfied with life and happy.

Let's use the example of moving to a new home to demonstrate how your lens on life can affect your happiness and satisfaction. Most people expect that moving will involve a lot of time and work and little fun. Let's assume that the rating for expectations is low (say, 4 on a scale of 1 to 10). But what is the perceived reality? Let's view the situation through two different lenses.

- **The negative lens:** "I am so overwhelmed by the fact that we have to move next month. How are we ever going to survive doing everything on our to-do list?" Perceived reality score? Low. (Let's assume a score of 3 on a scale of 1 to 10).
- **The positive lens:** "Moving next month will give our family an adventure and fresh perspective! We are going to have a lot of fun!" Perceived reality score? Higher. (Let's assume a score of 7 on a scale of 1 to 10).

We are viewing the exact same event, but in the first scenario, our perceived reality is low, so our satisfaction and happiness are negative. Mathematically, the situation translates as follows:

$$Satisfaction = Perceived\,Reality - Expectations$$
$$-1 = 3 - 4$$

In the second scenario, our perceived reality is higher, so our satisfaction and happiness are positive. Mathematically, the situation translates as follows:

$$Satisfaction = Perceived\,Reality - Expectations$$
$$3 = 7 - 4$$

See how the lens creates a completely different outcome for you and, likely, those around you? The move is either a "bummer" (-1) or "okay" (3) experience based on how you view it.

I love that *response* is part of the word *responsibility*. Know that you are responsible for your own responses to events; you cannot change other peoples' responses or actions. You can suggest a positive lens, but it is up to them to choose to use it and change their perspectives and, ultimately, their perceived realities. In her book, *Happy for No Reason*, Marci Shimoff writes about unconditional happiness. Using stories from her own life, as well as from the 100 people she interviewed, she shows how it is possible to be happy regardless of external circumstances. She demonstrates that it is not the size of your bank account or even the perfect mate that creates happiness. True happiness comes only from within.

Here's an exercise to help you manage your happiness and satisfaction. Start each day with:

"Thank you, Universe, for the great day coming up."

*Then, add your own details of how
you want the day to turn out.*

Before you go to bed at night, reflect on the day and find the positive things you experienced. If something didn't turn out the way you wanted, accept the possibility that the outcome was meant to be and that it can pave the way for something even greater. Then, as you are falling asleep, do this mental exercise:

"Thank you, Universe, for the great day you've given me."

Then, add your own details of why you are thankful.

Watch as your satisfaction and happiness grow over time.

SATISFACTION IS BASIC MATH.
MANAGE HAPPINESS ON YOUR LIFE PATH.

Putting a Positive Lens to the Test

Let's think back to the story of my consulting project with Frank, Alice, and Steve. After that fateful breakfast at the Holiday Inn, I set a new goal for my relationship with Alice: More satisfaction and happiness at work for both of us.

I began observing people at meetings to see if a positive or negative attitude played an important role or had any obvious effect on meeting outcomes. We consultants love correlations, often depicted as scatterplots, so I would jot down my observations on flights home. Over time, the correlation between attitudes and outcomes proved to be undeniable. As the consultant team's attitude improved from negative to positive, the client meeting outcomes improved. Conclusion: The attitude of our team was a critical element of our success.

Before every meeting, I started to preach the importance of our attitudes and smiles. Having a smile on was easy when flights arrived without delays, projects stayed on schedule, and the team and clients got along like old friends. But I reminded my consultants—and myself—that smiling in the face of duress was key. There were many times when I smiled on our way to a client meeting, despite a lack of sleep or lost baggage. I would remind my team and myself that *smiles beget success*. Bad attitudes and bemoaning situations out of our control lead to ruts and poor performance.

There was a pivotal moment within my unit when I knew that the *smiles beget success* lesson was fully integrated. It was about a year after our project with Frank and the blow-up at the Holiday Inn breakfast bar. We had spent the last year learning how to use *smile power* despite all odds. I finally felt that Alice was ready to deliver her first solo pitch, and I trusted her with a new client opportunity. The client's office was a few blocks away, so Alice's plan was to grab lunch in the café downstairs, spend some time preparing, and then walk over for the afternoon meeting. She gave herself plenty of time to ensure that she was completely ready when the presentation began.

I knew she would check in with me after the meeting, so I went through my email right before I left the office that evening. When I read her message, I doubled over with laughter and felt a sense of pride and relief.

TO: Kathryn

FROM: Alice

SENT: Mon 3/14/98 5:00PM CST

SUBJECT: meeting update

Hi. Update. Did you hear about the major elevator issue
in our building today? I was in the middle of it!

I was on my way down to grab a bite to eat when the
elevator jerked to a violent stop. The air conditioning
went off and everything went dark. You know I am not a
fan of enclosed places. Then the minutes—and then what
felt like hours—started to tick by! It was 300 degrees in
that elevator!

I started to freak out. Would I be late to the client
presentation? Would I boil in this dark inferno? Was
anyone coming for me? I started sweating like a
maniac. I think I almost had a panic attack!

Then I remembered what you have been saying,
"Smile, smile, smile." So I just started smiling and
pretending that I was already in the presentation,
doing a great job. Occasionally I would envision an
arctic breeze coming through to cool me down. The ·
sweat was pouring, but at least I was doing something
productive and imagining that I was comfortable.

Finally, the lights came on and the elevator jolted to a
start. The door opened and the maintenance guys stared
at me, hoping I was not going to come screaming out of
that hot prison. I realized it had only been 30 minutes,
not eight hours, but it was still a crazy journey. I walked

calmly to the ladies room and dried off the sweat.

I grabbed a smoothie on the way out since it was almost time for the meeting to start.

I got to the client building and prepared myself for the inevitable small talk.

"Good afternoon, Alice. How are you today?"

(Dramatic pause. Do I start off with my nightmare commute? No. Smile!)

"GREAT! THANKS!"

And we got straight to some really productive work.

You would have been proud. I think the meeting went extremely well, and they asked for a proposal. So, good news. Smiles beget success.

I will see you back in the office tomorrow morning.

Alice

OF HAPPINESS BE YOUR OWN CREATOR, EVEN WHEN YOU'RE STUCK IN THE ELEVATOR.

Mantra #1: Change your lens on life is a reminder that positivity can benefit you through many walks of life. Positivity can help you as you make major transitions, learn a new sport or skill, or struggle through work challenges. Smiling is an important component of positivity, as is body language. Remember how the Wonder Woman pose can reduce cortisol levels and increase testosterone. As Alice taught us, keeping a positive attitude even through challenging situations can increase the likelihood of success. Having a positive relationship with food is one of the best ways to establish healthy and balanced eating habits. *Change your lens on life* does not advocate putting on rose-colored glasses but instead taking a filtered view that magnifies the best of life.

ACTION ITEMS FROM THIS CHAPTER

FOR SUCCESS IN LIFE:

Know that your perspective shapes your reality. An optimistic lens can be most helpful during:

- **Transitions.** Make your decision, then make that decision the right decision. A smile will often seal the deal. Don't waste energy with what-ifs.
- **High-pressure events.** When you are scared or nervous, smiling will positively change your body chemistry, the tone of your voice, and the way others perceive you.
- **Challenging times.** Optimism will increase your chances of a successful outcome. Remember that when working with others, you get more with honey than with vinegar.

FOR SUCCESS IN WELLNESS:

- Remember that it is not just the food that you put on your plate that affects your wellness and energy levels. Evaluate your relationships, activities, and spiritual practices to get a more complete picture of how you nourish yourself.

- Avoid thinking about foods as bad versus good.
- Approach slow-down foods with moderation instead of making them taboo. Increase your intake of foods that make you go with energy.

Get Some Good Boots On

You can't build a great building on a
weak foundation. You must have a solid foundation
if you're going to have a strong superstructure.

—GORDON B. HINCKLEY
religious leader

In skiing, boots are arguably your most important piece of equipment. As the connection between you and your skis, boots should be thought of in the way that a general contractor thinks about the foundation of a house. Put well-constructed framing on top of a poorly laid foundation, and the result will be shaky. Build upon a strong and secure base, and what you put on top will be stronger and long lasting. In life, your foundation is a combination of education and experiences. Your wellness status, specifically your energy and stress levels, is integral to the strength of this base. Ultimately, your foundation gives you the expertise to take your game—be it at the office, on the playing field, or at home—to the next level.

A Love Story Almost Cut Short

The first time I had ventured into a ski town was in 1995 when I was 24. But before we get into that story, let's start with how I wound up there.

I met Jeff in 1994 at a wedding. I was a bridesmaid, and he was a groomsman. The bride, groom, and I had become friends as undergrads at Emory University. Their wedding was a huge event in Washington, D.C. at the National Cathedral. After several days of pre-parties and day and evening events, Jeff and I were inseparable. As the long weekend came to an end, Jeff borrowed his friend's car and drove me to the airport. Along the way, we made small talk, clearly trying to sneak in some of those key questions we all use as filters in the dating process:

- Anyone in your family marry a cousin?
- Spent much time in jail?
- Any violent tics or addictions?

Then came the bombshell from Jeff: "You *do* ski?" I remember the long, awkward silence that followed. I didn't know what to say. I had never lived near mountains. I attended college in Atlanta, Georgia and was a graduate student in Austin, Texas at the time.

The answer to break the uncomfortable silence: "Nope."

I remember watching a small, dark cloud of disappointment pass over Jeff's face. As I got out of the car at the airport, I felt a breeze, or maybe it was the early kiss of death to our relationship.

"I'll call you," said Jeff.

"Yeah. Talk to you later."

Surprisingly, Jeff overlooked the lack of ski experience, and we did talk—a lot. He was working on Wall Street, and I was in the second year of my MBA program. I was going through a stressful schedule of job interviews, traveling around the country for second or third rounds. A few of those trips sent me to New York, so I had a chance to see Jeff. He had no business in Austin, but he came anyway, and we enjoyed carefree weekends on Sixth Street. On one of those visits, the ski issue again reared its head.

"You really need to learn how to ski," Jeff said nonchalantly.

"Skiing is expensive, and I'm paying my way through graduate school here. I just don't know how that's going to work," I told him.

"Some friends of mine have a place in Sun Valley, and we're going to ski for a week this spring," Jeff said. "If you can get yourself a ticket, you should come and stay with us."

His face beamed with excitement, and I realized how important it was to him that I share in one of his favorite activities. "Sure, I'll think about it." I was committed to our relationship and realized that meant pushing myself out of my comfort zone so we could try new things together. After all, if Jeff loved skiing, how bad could it be?

The problem: Tickets from Austin to Sun Valley were probably about $1,000. Putting myself through business school meant I didn't have an extra grand sitting around.

Back at school the next week, a few friends and I were sitting in the student commons getting some homework done, when one of them said, "Hey, did you hear about the Finance Challenge coming up? A bunch of industry experts come in, give you a Harvard Business School case study, and ask you to solve it in 24 hours. You and your team come up with the best solution and then present your recommendation to a panel of experts."

"So, it's an invitation to stay up all night, argue in the group about the right answer, and then—once you feel death warming over because you haven't slept and have been debating all night—stand up in front of an audience that can't wait to fillet and grill you alive?" I joked.

"But the winning team members get a thousand bucks each."

Cha-ching. I thanked the universe in advance for allowing me to win the Finance Challenge.

It was one of the most difficult 24 hours of my young life. I ended up on a great team, but we were challenged to find a unified strategy, and we struggled until the wee hours to compromise on a solution to the case study that we were willing to present to the panel of judges. We barely got our slides ready in time for our first-round presentation, and by then I was so tired that my amygdala, the part of the brain that controls emotion, was starting to override my frontal lobe, which manages executive function.

I blew it as I stumbled in a daze through the main parts of my presentation, but I reached deep down for strength during the question and answer sessions and knocked the ball out of the park with my responses to tough questions. Though I felt somewhat humiliated by my subpar performance, we ultimately won. After a good long cry of relief and the longest nap of my life, I awoke to the realization that I had secured my path to becoming a skier.

PREPARE THE FOUNDATION,
EVEN THROUGH DEGRADATION
AND SLEEP DEPRIVATION.

All I Really Need to Know I Learned in Romper Room?

It was spring break, and I had arrived in Sun Valley to meet up with Jeff and his buddies from Wall Street. As we talked over breakfast about the upcoming day, I got the sense that I was the only one new to the sport.

> "Can't wait to hit the moguls!"
> "I hope we get some powder while we're here!"
> "I'm going to hit the NASTAR racing course!"

After we had gotten our rental ski equipment in order, it was time to hit the slopes, and I was looking forward to my first lesson. I soon learned that, in Sun Valley, beginners don't even go to the same mountain as the more experienced skiers. I was the only one staying at the beginner hill, Dollar Mountain.

"See ya!" Jeff and his friends shouted as the huge Suburban they had rented pulled away. I was left behind and alone, and I looked around to see that I was standing in the middle of a sea of tiny heads no higher than my waistline. They were swarming about in huge masses, and there was a lot of noise.

Have I been left in ski school for kids?

I won't go into all of the humbling details of my first day in ski school, including sitting at a lunch table eating peanut butter and jelly sandwiches while runny noses dripped all over the placemats, or how there were sing-song times, tiny cubbies, and a reading circle. I was learning how to ski with the four-year-olds. I guess I really wanted to learn.

FORTIFY THE FOUNDATION,
EVEN THROUGH BOOGERS AND ISOLATION.

Confidence from the Ground Up

I asked my instructor, Parker, what it would take for me to graduate to the big mountain, Baldy. After all, from the kiddie hill, I could see that life over at Baldy was looking pretty good. I learned that the end of the ski day is appropriately called *après ski*, which involves people sitting around, tanning, drinking beer, and relaxing. No boogers anywhere to be seen.

"You have to be able to get down the steeps and have confidence that you won't get stuck in a place where you can't get down safely. It doesn't require expert technique," he assured me. "But you have to start with your feet."

"Can you show me how?" I asked.

For the rest of the afternoon we worked on a confidence-building drill called side-slipping. It is a great technique in case you get to a slope that looks too steep, icy, bumpy, or creepy—whatever gets you nervous on your skis. At that point, you just side-slip down, slowly, until you get to a spot on the mountain that looks friendlier. Then, you start your turns. The trick to doing the drill correctly is that you really need to focus on your feet.

Side-slipping teaches you that skiing starts inside your boots. Movement in side-slipping starts exactly when you roll your ankles downhill and take the pressure off the edges of your skis. You are doing nothing else with your body—your upper half and even your legs are steady, and you are getting down the mountain safely. Most importantly, the drill builds confidence that you can get down anything—even the big mountain.

By the end of the week, I had done so much work on my feet that my toes were aching. I have different sized feet (by a size and a half!), and I had decided to go with a ski boot that fit the smaller foot. The extra tightness on my large foot became unbearable.

"Man, my feet are killing me!" I exclaimed as we sat around the *après ski* table (*sans* boogers).

"They are supposed to!" all the Wall Streeters said in unison.

"Really? Why?" I wondered.

"You have to wear those boots *tight*, my friend," one of the expert skiers added. "It's the only way to be one with your skis."

As I learned more about skiing, I came to agree that a good boot fit is key, but it shouldn't be painful. Back at Dollar, the thrill of having built a foundation in skiing during that week of ski school overwhelmed the pain, but on the plane ride home to Austin, I reveled in the relief of my gym shoes. Later that year, even after one toenail on my larger foot had turned black and finally fallen off, I was still thrilled with what I had learned on my ski vacation at Sun Valley. And I was hooked!

KNOW THAT YOU CAN PREVAIL,
EVEN IF YOU LOSE A TOENAIL.

Breakfast: Build Your Foundation for Each and Every Day

"Gotta start your day with breakfast!" my dad, Dr. Robert Kemp, cheerfully reminded us as he woke my sister and me in our hotel room.

As a biochemist, my dad ("Dr. Bob") frequently spoke at conferences around the world. My sister and I were always thrilled when he allowed us to tag along, mostly because we loved to lounge at the hotel pool. When we were teenagers, he had a conference in Puerto Rico during one of many long and frigid Chicago winters, so we begged him to let us come. He relented on the condition that we would not sleep until noon, as usual, but instead enjoy the fresh air and maybe even the historical sites. And, of course, we also had to listen to his biochemist views at mealtime.

"Protein makes up the building blocks of your body," he pontificated as we made our way down the hall to the breakfast room. "Breakfast is the meal of champions," he continued.

So we made sure to get all of our macronutrients and as many micronutrients as we could at the breakfast bar. My dad was a sucker for Canadian bacon, which they offered in stacks at the hotel, so he was definitely going to get his protein.

As we sat down to eat, my sister asked my dad, "How many people are you speaking to today?"

"About a thousand," my dad answered. "So I'd better make sure that I don't have anything stuck in my teeth before I start." He dabbed his napkin against his professor-like face and looked at us in a very serious, ivory-tower way. Then, he took a bite of his beloved Canadian bacon. There was a disturbing CRACK noise. His eyes grew wide, and he panicked as he looked around for his napkin. He stooped below the table and, as inconspicuously as possible, spit something into his napkin. When he sat upright again, he looked straight at my sister and me.

Gasp!

Having something stuck in his teeth was the *least* of my dad's worries. At the front of his smile sat an enormous black hole. He had just chipped off a huge chunk of his front tooth.

"Cool, Dad! You look just like Wayne Gretzky!" I said admiringly.

My dad looked at Suzanne, who had burst into an uncontrolled laugh.

"No, you look like Billy Bob!" Suzanne managed to say through her tears of laughter.

My dad was getting flustered. His talk was in 15 minutes. There was simply nothing he could do. He would have to make his keynote presentation as Dr. Billy Bob.

START YOUR DAY WITH A GREAT MEAL,
EVEN IF IT ENDS WITH BILLY BOB APPEAL.

How to Break the Fast, Not Your Tooth

Breakfast literally means *break the fast*. To fast is to go without food for more than eight hours. Your body does this every night, assuming you don't raid the fridge at midnight, so it is important to fuel up in the morning before you set off on your busy day. Without breakfast, you might start to feel sluggish or even get the shakes.

Remember laying the foundation? Breakfast can help you focus on your work and be more successful, whether that means better performance at school, increased productivity at work, or more positivity as a family and community member.

Here are some top reasons to eat breakfast:

• Breakfast gives your body energy and much-needed nutrients after the fast. Kids and adults who eat breakfast perform better in sports. The theory is that breakfast-skippers might not be getting the vitamins, minerals, and other nutrients they need.
• Breakfast starts up your metabolism in the morning, helping you to maintain a healthy weight. Getting into a meal routine helps to keep your appetite under control. Breakfast eaters are less likely to overeat at other meals or snacks.
• Meals in the morning can help to put you in a happier mood!

Breakfast should be made up of the following key components, listed here in order of importance:

1. **A protein source.** Dr. Billy Bob's advice was accurate. Protein provides the building blocks for our bodies. Without it, we can't sustain our strength. Always remember your protein.
2. **A fruit or vegetable.** We need to get at least five servings of fruits and vegetables every day, so why not start in the morning? Fruits and vegetables provide so many great nutrients— and are so delicious—it's important not to miss out.

3. **Whole grains.** Note the word "whole." The advice to eat whole grains does not mean a white bagel or toast before you run out the door. If that's all you eat, you are likely to be out of energy and really hungry in an hour or two. Whole grains include all parts of the grain and are minimally processed, so your body will take its time converting them to energy. The new MyPlate (USDA nutrition guidelines) tells us that half our grains should be whole, but I think the more the better. Whole grains include oatmeal, barley, quinoa, millet, brown rice, bulgur wheat, and many others.

4. **A healthy fat.** Add healthy oils, like olive oil, nuts, or avocado to your breakfast. Fats take a while to digest, so they keep you full longer. Fats have all kinds of good things in them like omega-3 fatty acids, the helpful kind that help to build a healthy brain. A simple trick to getting those omega-3s is to sprinkle ground flax seeds on anything you prepare. This addition is a nice way to change it up if you don't feel like adding olive oil, nut butter, or large seeds to your meal. (Note: Store ground flax seeds in the freezer, as they are particularly sensitive to becoming rancid.)

How do you include all four of these components when you prepare a great breakfast in your own home? Here are ten ideas for a yummy, healthy, and sustaining breakfast to get you started.

1. A hard-boiled egg, buttered whole-grain toast
   (sprinkled with ground flax seeds, if you like),
   and a pear.

2. Oatmeal with cherries, raisins, honey, and almonds.

3. Brown rice with avocado and pepper with an egg on top.

4. A smoothie containing fruit, nut butter, and oatmeal (soak oatmeal overnight in milk).

5. Steel-cut oats with nut butter (thin with milk, if necessary) stirred in. Add a little honey for sweetness. Mix in apple slices or enjoy them on the side.

6. Homemade pancakes/waffles. (Try my recipe for protein pancakes, which uses eggs, ricotta cheese, and whole-grain flour.*) Serve grapes on the side.

7. Scrambled eggs with chunks of roasted butternut squash and cheese.

8. Nitrate-free turkey rolls, cheese slices, Triscuits, and apples (my daughter's go-to when we are running late).

9. Nut butter and jelly sandwich on whole-grain bread with apple slices (my son's go-to when we are running late).

10. Whole-grain tortilla with nut butter, banana, and raisins.

Use fruits and vegetables, whole-grain and protein sources, and seasonings that your family enjoys.

KNOW THE RIGHT WAY
TO STRUCTURE THE FIRST MEAL OF YOUR DAY.

---

* For the protein pancake recipe, visit www.healthykidsideas.com and type "protein pancakes" into the search box on the sidebar on the right hand side. Or search "breakfast" for many additional ideas.

Breakfast For Non-Morning People

You know it's important to eat a healthy breakfast, yet sometimes you just don't make the time for it. Here's a short list to follow to make sure that you always break the fast in a healthy way.

- *Make it available* by putting healthy choices in your refrigerator and on your shelves.
- *Plan ahead* by using the night before to set out dishes, cut up fruits and vegetables, and so on. If you have kids, know that they will be more likely to enjoy breakfast if they are contributing to the planning and preparation.
- *Make it easy* by preparing your own grab-and-go breakfasts for the days that you have little time to sit down to eat. You can pre pack your healthy breakfasts into small containers and freeze or refrigerate them.
- *Use a rice cooker* to make hot breakfasts that are simple and nutritious. Instructions are coming up next.

DON'T WORRY IF YOUR DAY STARTS SLOW.
USE TIME-SAVING TIPS THAT YOU KNOW.

Can One Common Appliance Replace All Your Cookbooks?

Embrace flexibility when cooking based on your personal taste, your budget, and what you happen to have on hand. In other words, don't get too caught up following recipes. Recipes are great for learning how to cook or learning how to combine food elements. And, of course, recipes are essential to baking because making cakes, cookies, and pastries is more of a science.

But cooking is an art, and you need to embrace your inner artist when you are in the kitchen. I am going to reveal the art of cooking a delicious, nutritious, warm breakfast with ease by using a Recipe Framework. But first things first: Let's unravel the mystery of the rice cooker.

This little powerhouse of a cooking appliance is the victim of the worst product-naming snafu in the history of devices. Why? Because most people who happen to own a rice cooker think to use it only when they are making rice.

Big mistake!

My rice cooker sits on the counter as a most honored guest in my kitchen. In the spirit of its Japanese heritage, I've renamed my rice cooker *cooker-san,* or most honored cook. Many college students can tell you how to make everything from sautéed salmon (which I've done and enjoyed) to BBQ ribs (which I have not tried) in a rice cooker; however, it is whole grains, lentils, and split peas that follow the exact same rules as rice. There's no guessing and no slaving over the stove, watching pots that boil (or don't, according to the old adage). The cooker-san does everything for you, independent of your watchful eye!

Here are the simple steps to becoming friends with your own cooker-san*:

STEP 1: Rinse the grains/lentils/split peas to remove dust and other particles. Grains can also be soaked overnight, making them easier to digest. If you decide to soak

* For ideas on what type of rice cooker to purchase, visit www.
healthysolutionsofsv.com and click on "Recommended Products"
on the green navigation bar.

them, you can add a little lemon juice because the acid helps break them down even more.

STEP 2: Measure using the 2:1 rule. For every cup of grains/lentils/split peas, put in two cups of water.

STEP 3: Press down the on button. It will shift to the warm position when the grains/lentils/split peas are done.

STEP 4: Unplug it once the rice cooker clicks to warm. If you are a lazy cook like me, you can also leave the pot sitting there for a while on warm. Then, you are ready to make something yummy with your grains/lentils/split peas. Note that, when cooked, all three expand to two to three times their dry size.

STEP 5: Dress up those cooker-san goodies. It's time to break your reliance on recipes! When I want to plan a meal quickly and simply, I avoid cookbooks like the plague. My worst fear is that the recipe will call for an ingredient that I don't have (or recognize), and then we will have a dreaded extra trip to the grocery store. When I need to be an efficient cook (which is 99% of the time), I avoid complex recipes and long shopping lists and instead think about a meal in terms of a Recipe Framework. Recipe Frameworks give you a basic understanding of what elements you might like to combine (for example, a grain with a protein source, some vegetables, a healthy fat, and seasonings) to make a delicious, nutritious meal. Recipe Frameworks allow you to make the decisions about what goes into your dish based on your family's food preferences as well as what you have on hand in your fridge, freezer, and pantry. Recipe Frameworks make healthy meal planning flexible, simple, and easy.

In 2008, Nurture created a set of Recipe Frameworks, including the Grain Recipe Framework for Breakfasts. We also created Recipe Frameworks for lunches and dinners, bean dips, soups, and breakfast smoothies*. We found that these recipes were life changers for so many people, empowering them to start cooking and get back into the kitchen. As a smaller nonprofit organization operating in only two states, Nurture was thrilled that the national organization Share our Strength's Cooking Matters adopted our Recipe Frameworks concept and has, in turn, reached hundreds of thousands of people.

Breakfast Recipe Framework

Whole Grain (Cooked)	+	Protein/ Fat Source	+	Seasoning(s)	+	Fruit
oatmeal		yogurt		honey		apple slices
quinoa		cottage cheese		cinnamon		berries
buckwheat		nuts		nutmeg		bananas
millet		flax seeds		etc.		cherries
rice		other seeds				mango
barley		cooked eggs				peaches
etc.		etc.				raisins
						etc.

* To see all of the Recipe Frameworks, please visit www.nurtureyourfamily.org and click on "Cooking Class Resources" on the blue navigation bar. Scroll down to "Recipe Frameworks".

MAKE COOKING EASY WITH RECIPE FRAMEWORKS.
YOU WILL BENEFIT FROM THE MANY PERKS.

Avoid the Great White Hazards

Sugary cereals and the white breakfast foods, such as bagels, English muffins, and croissants, do not build the proper foundation for your day. These common breakfast foods cause a spike in your blood sugar and then a huge drop, leaving you feeling hungry and tired by mid-morning.

Dr. Maria Maricich, Functional Medicine Doctor and Light Touch Chiropractor in Ketchum, Idaho and a former U.S. Olympic downhill ski racer once ranked tenth in the world, believes that blood sugar fluctuations are one of the root causes of our society's health decline, including reduced brain function. Maricich likens rapid blood sugar fluctuations to taking your car and revving it up (high blood sugar) and then slamming on the brakes (low blood sugar). Over time, the result is a worn-out car or a worn-out body.

Just as a house built on a shaky foundation will fall down over time, a body running on inadequate nutrition, especially at the start of the day, will fall apart over time.

WHITE FOODS TO START YOUR DAY
WILL SEND THE DOCTOR YOUR WAY.

The Price of Mastery

It takes time for a proper foundation to be dug, poured, and backfilled. It must then cure and harden, a process that cannot be rushed. In the same way, we cannot rush our success in life, including in our careers.

After graduate school, I started my career with grand ideas of running meetings, entertaining happy clients, and celebrating unbridled success. What I learned was, as with anything else in life, things rarely come easily or right away. I put in long hours looking at enormous databases and doing much of the work that the more senior folks in our firm simply didn't want to do. It was time to pay my dues and put in the sweat-equity that is necessary to be successful in any career or endeavor.

In her book *This Isn't the Life I Ordered*, Jen Weigel, an Emmy Award-winning reporter and advocate of positive news, discusses the importance of never allowing our egos to tell us we are too good for any task or job. Who is to say that we are above what might seem like menial or entry-level work? If you have seen the movie *The Karate Kid*, remember how Daniel (played by Ralph Macchio) was pretty annoyed when he showed up for his special training in martial arts with Mr. Miyagi (Pat Morita) and ended up washing cars and painting fences. In one iconic scene, Daniel waxed a long line of cars as Mr. Miyagi had him repeat a simple phrase as he went through the repetitive motions: "Wax on. Wax off. Wax on. Wax off." By the end of the movie, we learn the method to Miyagi's madness. These incredibly simple tasks had built up a system of reflexes, balance, and agility that allowed Daniel to win the karate tournament.

When we are building a foundation, we must be open to any possibility. You never know what you might learn or who you might meet if you are open to trying new things.

As a college student, I took a summer internship with the State of Illinois in a position that offered opportunities to work in various areas of government. I was stationed primarily in the office of cultural affairs, where my fellow intern buddy, Ximena, and I wrote captions for pictures on news releases related to consular outreach efforts and cultural groups. We were assigned to the State of Illinois Center building in Chicago, where Governor Jim Edgar had an office on the same floor. The governor was not in Chicago often, as he was primarily based in Springfield, the state capital. Nonetheless, Ximena and I were constantly on the lookout for a chance encounter with this important and charismatic politician. Quite often, we ran into one of his assistants, Ana Maria, who managed Governor Edgar's schedule and sorted letters he received from constituents. Ana Maria was from South America and had the most beautiful accent. She had a unique way of saying words that began with the letter s, always adding an *eh* sound to the beginning. I could always tell when she came down the hall to talk to someone in our department. I listened closely to, and with admiration of, her captivating accent as I drank my morning tea.

"I have a very eh-special job down at the governor's office. Very eh special, indeed. I don't eh-suppose you might have eh-someone that might be able to come and work in the governor's eh-suite this afternoon?" she asked our manager one morning.

"Sure. We have those two interns, Kathryn and Ximena. They are college students and have pretty good writing skills. We've been increasing their responsibility level each week, and they always keep up."

"They would be eh-super."

"Great. They will *love* the opportunity to work for the governor's office. Why don't I lend them to you when you need them?"

"Eh-sounds good."

We were summoned that very afternoon. Ximena and I had spent our lunch break dreaming about the exciting projects we might work on. Would we do research? Help with a news release? Provide our insights on how to charm the younger generation at the next election? The governor might even be there, and we dreamed he would see how smart we were and would ask us to come work for him directly!

As we went into the office, our anticipation was high. The office was actually a suite of rooms, decked out in expensive-looking furniture. There was a dining room, small living room, and other rooms we couldn't see. Everything was quiet and dark, and our hopes sank—the governor wasn't there. Ana Maria didn't show us around too much as she led us to an area with lots of gleaming and fancy china on display. Ximena and I oohed and aahed at how pretty everything was and, after a somewhat awkward silence, Ana Maria turned to leave. She looked back at us as if to say we should eh-stay where we were.

"You will be eh-spending your time here," Ana Maria said as she gestured toward the huge china cabinets and handed us each a dust rag. "Everything is very ... how do you say? *With dust.*"

Then she walked away while Ximena and I looked at each other, our mouths gaping. We slowly came to the realization that we were on "eh-special assignment" as the governor's maid service. I took the dust rag and thought of Daniel in *The Karate Kid*.

Wax on. Wax off. Wax on. Wax off. Wax on. Wax off.

Ximena and I dusted that china until it gleamed. We had fun and laughed and told jokes while we worked. The governor never showed up, but a young speechwriter stopped by the office and poked his head in to see what we were laughing about.

"Hey, what are you guys doing in here?"

"We're interns."

"Doin' the dishes, eh?" he mused.

"You bet," we smiled back.

A week later, we received an invitation to a photo shoot* with the governor himself:

> You guys did such a great job on the china,
> we wanted to thank you.
> —Chief Speech Writer,
> Office of the Governor of Illinois

PAYING YOUR DUES IS KEY,
JUST LIKE IN THE KARATE KID MOVIE.

---

* To see the photo, visit www.healthysolutionsofsv.com/
political-pictures/

Pouring the Foundation, Wall Street Style

Wall Street is infamous for asking its entry-level workers to pay their dues. In *Outliers,* author Malcolm Gladwell says that it takes roughly 10,000 hours of practice to achieve mastery in a field. The average full-time job requires about 2,000 hours per year. That means that you become an expert in roughly five years. Based on the stories Jeff would share with me about his rat-race days in New York's financial district, I surmise that a Wall Street strategy is to create experts in a year or less; all you have to do is work new hires five times as hard as the average person!

Jeff and his colleagues were typically assigned a huge workload around 5 p.m. and expected to have an extraordinary amount of progress turned in by the next morning. Working all night was the norm, and sometimes it turned into a strange form of mental torture. The infamous all-nighters often left behind a trail of emails such as this one.

TO: Jeffrey
FROM: Sina
SENT: Tues 3/12/96 3:04AM EST
SUBJECT: This sucks

Jeff,

It's 3:00 in the morning.

I'm not going home any time soon.

I spent the entire weekend in the office.

I'm tired, I'm cold, and I'm hungry.

And there are wolves after me.

This sucks.

Later,

STG

On other days, the long hours and intensity of the job rendered these highly educated but over-taxed workers a little punchy and creative.

TO: Jeffrey

FROM: James

SENT: Mon 6/9/97 11:26AM EST

SUBJECT: Neruda in person

The machine purrs out the pages like gentle waves
in Ecuador,
I caress these pages, knowing their power, their saucy
truculence
–A Cuban flower girl;
These pages hold my truth, my damnation.
O mysterious Love, I know you
–Your name is EBITDA.
Pablo Neruda

My point in sharing these silly, pathetic, and absolutely true emails is to show that it is okay to work yourself to the point when you can't remember what country a famous poet comes from or when you believe you are being hunted by wolves in a busy metropolitan city. Working yourself past the point of comfort is part of achieving success in any career and in many worthwhile endeavors in life. Paying your dues is part of mastering your trade and succeeding. It's worth it.

SOLIDIFY YOUR BASE,
EVEN IN THE RAT RACE.

Mantra #2: Get some good boots on is a reminder that building a strong foundation in life and health should be a top priority. Skiing reminds us that our success is built from the bottom up, starting with our feet. A solid foundation in life is built through education and experiences. We should be open to the possibility of growth, even through what may seem like the most mundane tasks, as we learned from my experience in the governor's office.

You have the opportunity to strengthen your foundation each and every day, starting with a great breakfast. Just like Dr. Billy Bob teaches, include protein along with whole grains, healthy fats, and fruits or veggies. Use the Nurture Recipe Frameworks to create delicious and nutritious breakfasts that are low-cost, easy to prepare, and time-efficient.

ACTION ITEMS FROM THIS CHAPTER

FOR SUCCESS IN LIFE:

- Thank the universe in advance for what you need. A thousand bucks for a plane ticket is just a starting point in terms of what an appreciated universe can provide. Understand the law of attraction.

- Practice. Be prepared. Do your homework. Put in the hours you need when you are learning something new. It takes 10,000 hours of committed time to master any skill.
- Pay your dues and know that any suffering is only temporary. In Mantra #4 (Plant Your Poles), we'll discuss the principle that life is long. There is plenty of time later in life to sit in the hot tub.

FOR SUCCESS ON THE SLOPES:

- Never assume that you are a better skier than the four-year-olds. They are closer to the ground, so falling doesn't hurt as much.
- Remember that skiing starts with your feet.
- Side-slip to build your confidence before you hit the bigger slopes.

FOR SUCCESS IN WELLNESS:

- Eat breakfast every day. Know why it's important and know how to create simple and healthy options.
- Involve your inner cooking artist by using the Recipe Frameworks. For maximum efficiency and ease, try a rice cooker, or *cooker-san.*
- Put in the long hours when you need to but recognize that the stories of all-nighters at work involved folks in their 20s and 30s. Always keep balance in mind for optimal wellness.

Zoom Out for the Best View

You have to participate relentlessly
in the manifestation of your own blessings.

—ELIZABETH GILBERT

author and 2015 Sun Valley Wellness Festival keynote speaker

When we moved to Sun Valley, I hadn't even heard of backcountry skiing, but I soon learned how different it was from resort skiing. Backcountry skiers tackle runs that can't be reached by ski lifts. Some take helicopters to the top of a peak, while others "earn their turns" by climbing the mountain themselves. In addition to avoiding lift lines, these skiers are rewarded with untouched powder and a pristine landscape. I gained an appreciation for those folks who had already had their workout by the time they reached the top of the mountain, as opposed to people like me, who relax on the way up by taking the chairlift. No matter which route you choose, once you get to the mountaintop, the change in perspective is undeniable. Skiing offers ongoing opportunities for zooming in and zooming out, for seeing the forest and seeing the trees. It provides countless chances to cultivate vision, see the big picture, and work on visualization, manifesting reality through mental exercise.

I Am a Great Monkey

While I enjoyed nearly every moment of my time with the DIVAS grandmas, by Year 2 of the program, in the 2012-13 winter season, I was ready to move up. I fit in with a much more aggressive group and first experienced the challenge and excitement of running gates, skiing as fast as you can around flags in a predefined S-line, as they do in the giant slalom in the Olympics. While learning to run gates with the DIVAS, I also first experienced the power of visualization in sports.

"We are going to first just slowly slip through the course so you know where you are going," said Nicky, the amazing red-coated ski instructor. "Then, we go back up, muster up your courage and go again. Only faster." Nicky gave us one of her famous smiles that said, *"Come on,* I know you can do it!"

We took turns going down through the course, which was getting icy, making it hard to stay in control. Not what I would call *hero snow* conditions. We were doing terribly, and Tanya, one of my group members, bashed into a set of gates. She limply waved goodbye at the bottom of the course, yelling up before she left, "I think I need to go get this X-rayed. See you next week, I hope".

Gloom and doom fell over the group. Nicky picked up on it right away, perhaps because no one volunteered to ski next.

"Okay. New approach!" she yelled with encouragement. "Have you ever heard about visualization practices that Olympians use?"

A few, but not all, of our helmeted heads nodded.

"You simply visualize your successful run through the course, completing it all in your head before you actually do it physically."

We all looked at her quizzically, not sure how this was going to prevent trips to the hospital for our own sets of X-rays.

Nicky knew she had to keep it simple for us. "Okay. Never mind the entire process of visualization. Have you all heard of Muhammad Ali, the famous boxer?"

All of our helmets went up and down in unison.

"He would say to himself, over and over before he entered the ring, 'I am the greatest.' I want you all to do that now and then try the course again." Nicky smiled at us with encouragement. We followed her down the course again, this time much faster. My gut was twisting with fear, so I tried to keep those words of encouragement from the famous boxer in my heart and my mind.

I am the greatest. I am the greatest. I am the greatest.

Over the next hour, we did short loops through the course to get as much practice as possible. Going through the gates again and again, while still frightening, was becoming almost tedious. To change it up, every once in a while, I would replace the Muhammad Ali chant with "monkey visualize, monkey do!" It was a spin on the "monkey see, monkey do" phrase that had always made me smile. These tactics, with Nicky's encouragement, helped me get past my fear and start having some fun.

Even now, whenever I see gates, a chorus starts in my head: *I am the greatest. Monkey visualize, monkey do. I am the greatest.*

Later that week, while on a dinner date with Jeff, I asked him if he had any experience with visualization at work.

"You mean before a big presentation for a client?" he asked.

"Yes. For example, do you and your colleagues first visualize that the meeting will go well to give yourselves a boost in that positive direction?"

"No way. It's usually a kick in the pants about something or other, or nothing at all, before we go into a meeting."

Hmm. I guess that positive visualization still might be a little too woo-woo (my affectionate term for anything that might be considered alternative or complementary science and medicine) for the Wall Street types, but Jeff did like the greatest monkey story.

MANIFEST FROM HEART AND MIND.
BE THE GREATEST MONKEY OF YOUR KIND.

Free Throws, Olympians, and Dry iPhones

It turns out that visualization is not woo-woo at all. It is actually an important mental rehearsal that most professional athletes use regularly. The effectiveness of visualization has been studied rigorously and goes well beyond anecdotal references. In one study from the 1960s, Professor L.V. Clark of Wayne State University showed that high school basketball players were able to improve their free-throw shooting with *mental exercise* alone. One can only imagine the amazing things that can result from a combination of visualization and quality physical practice.

Most of us agree that being an Olympian is a pretty amazing feat. When I had the opportunity to interview cross-country skier Liz Stephen, a two-time U.S. Olympian, I asked about her mental exercise routines. "Visualization is actually *really* hard," Liz said. "It is an art to get it just right. You can't stop with simply seeing the course and how you will successfully navigate it. You have to actually *feel* it. It is a visceral thing. Feeling that success, for me, is key."

Liz helped me understand that visualization is not simply imagining you are watching yourself from the third-person perspective in a movie. While it should involve mental imagery, visualization also relies on seeing the actions from your first-person viewpoint, as though you are actually doing them. It involves sound and, most importantly, feeling. Unlike watching a movie, visualization becomes a vivid experience in which you have complete control over a successful performance and finish with a firm belief. These techniques can be used to create mental awareness, a sense of well-being, and confidence. The time I spent talking with Liz left me feeling light, buoyant, and infused with the possibility of what great things we all can achieve with a little vision and visualization.

That light feeling of possibility lasted until I attended the Dent conference a few days later. The event focused on the high tech industry but targeted all individuals interested in "making a dent in the universe." The conference itself and the speakers were great, but the scene in the lobby and the folks walking around during the breaks had me worried. They were all hunched over their phones, oblivious to who and what was around them. These were high-powered individuals capable of manifesting great things in this world, and they had paid great sums to come to Sun Valley and network with others. How could they have vision when they were hunched over their smartphones and tablets, tap-tap-tapping like squirrels frantically trying to open a nut?

The scene reminded me of a video my son had recently shown me of a man walking through a pool area. The man was so engrossed in an animated conversation on his iPhone that he walked right into the water. My son thought it was hilarious, but I thought it was representative and scary. People can become so engaged in multi-tasking that they can lose sight of the bigger picture.

I went back inside to the conference room to learn that one of the afternoon speakers was one of my favorite political cartoonists, David Horsey of the *Los Angeles Times*. In his session, he talked about some of his favorite drawings. The highlight for me was his cartoon "The Evolution of Man," which depicts a man walking along a mural of life-sized figures illustrating the various stages of human evolution, from ape to homo erectus to homo sapiens. The man happens to be lined up with these other figures as if he would be the next stage of mankind. The scary part is that he is shown as a step back in evolution, hunched over his phone. I thought to myself:

Yes, we have got to look up and have some vision, or we are headed for trouble indeed.

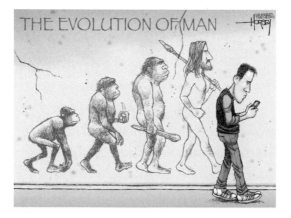

MANIFEST FROM HEART AND MIND.
DON'T GO BACKWARDS AS MANKIND.

Mindfulness As a Tool for Vision and Visualization

"What would you recommend to someone who is thinking about trying out meditation as a starting point?" I was interviewing Ryan Redman, co-founder of the Flourish Foundation and an expert on mindfulness practices, during an episode of "Healthy Kids Corner," my radio show on KDPI FM Ketchum Community Radio. I was expecting him to answer with one of the action steps that get someone to sit his or her butt down on a meditation cushion and just get to it.

Instead, his response surprised me.

"Step one is not so much clearing the mind but, instead, really taking the time to consider and reflect upon the benefits of developing these qualities of the mind."

You mean you don't want me to go out and buy a meditation cushion right away?

"If we don't seriously consider the impact the mind is having on us on a daily basis, then all the other priorities will take over," Ryan said. "So, for most people, a good place to start is to envision what it would be like to act from a place of mindfulness."

Okay folks, don't run out to buy a meditation chime alarm yet.

Ryan suggested we first ask questions like:

- What if I had the ability to make a conscious choice about what type of thoughts I'm going to enact through my behavior and speech?
- What would it be like if I weren't running from one thing to the next, always feeling overwhelmed?
- How would it feel to show up knowing that I have the inner resources to work skillfully with whatever is presented?

- What would it be like to act from a place that is grounded, contained, present, and aware?
- How would this vision affect me personally?
- What would be the ripple effect in other areas of my life and for other people?

"If we can reflect on these questions clearly, then, naturally, we will be motivated to put aside the time to create a mindfulness practice," Ryan continued wisely.

No wonder I have always considered Ryan to be our local mindfulness Jedi.

We then talked about the alternative to this vision of mindfulness, which is when your thoughts start to take over like a jail riot. One rumination arises after another, and then another appears with a vengeance. Do you have the capacity to choose whether this series of thoughts is truly beneficial or not? Unlikely!

There is a benefit to having spontaneous thoughts, but there are also many thoughts that are not relevant or are destructive to well-being. Controlling the jail riot in your mind means creating some space in between thoughts. To do that, you must recognize and *observe* your thoughts. We must create a gap between the stimulus and response to make room for choice in between.

After the interview with Ryan, I went home to spend an afternoon with my kids. I was thinking about the jail riot analogy as I sat in Elena's room while she moved around to attend to her various pets. From her desk came an incessant squeak creak, squeak creak. It was her hamster, Bobo, as she spun relentlessly on her wheel. While I was glad that Bobo was getting some exercise, I started to feel bad for her as she spun around and around, going nowhere. It was almost as if she was possessed as she put one little pink paw in front of the other. She was on a mission, with a vengeance.

Did she have any idea where she was going? Why she was running with such agitation? Was she even making a choice?

I thought to myself: As we go through life, considering our thoughts about our overall health, we don't want to be hamsters on a wheel.

VISUALIZE WHERE YOU WANT TO GO.
DON'T SPIN ON A WHEEL LIKE BOBO.

Your Vision Is What Leads the Way

"Chin up!" reminded Claudia, the day's inspiring ski instructor. We were on the slopes on a beautiful blue-sky day.

"Your body goes where you're looking. Why are you looking down at your ski tips?" she asked me.

She was right. I realized that I had been looking at my skis to check the distance between them. I had been guilty of crossing my skis, a much-hated move that never ends well, and I definitely didn't want to do it again.

"Focus ahead. Eyes up!" she encouraged me.

I thought about the concept of *drishti* in my yoga practice. Drishti is the ability to control and direct the focus, first of the eyes and then of the attention. Drishti assists concentration, aids movement, and allows us to orient our bodies. I realized that if I applied drishti to skiing, I would become more aware of the placement of my limbs and equipment automatically, without actually having to look at them. On the way down, I fell once, landing right on my butt, but I picked myself up and focused for the rest of my descent.

When I reached the bottom of the hill, I stopped to look around me. Oh, the beauty of the day! The wind blew on my cheeks, and I admired the view of infinity as I looked out to the mountain peaks in the far distance. Why had I limited myself to staring at my skis? How could I possibly miss the majesty of nature all around me?

"Take in the bigger picture and enjoy the scenery at the mountaintop," said Claudia. "Savor the great views while you're on the lift. But when you're coming down, keep your attention focused ahead of you and lead with your head and upper body pointing in the direction that you want to go."

"Your gaze also helps with your balance," she said to me with a smile and a wink. I guess she had seen me take that huge wipeout a few minutes earlier.

HAVE VISION AND DON'T BE BLIND.
KEEP FROM FALLING ON YOUR BEHIND.

Start by Asking Why

As we got on the next lift, one of my ski buddies turned to me and said, "You know, it's important to remember why we come up here week after week, trying to improve our skills. I come to get my workout in. What motivates you?"

I took a deep breath and thought this question through. I wasn't really skiing for the workout, because you spend a lot of time sitting on lifts and learning technique through drills, instruction, and discussion. If I wanted a workout, lacing up my running shoes and hitting the trails for 45 minutes would be a lot more efficient. Then, I thought about the scene I encountered when I first arrived at the lodge at the base of the mountain. In one area, families cooperated to get their ski gear in order as they eagerly anticipated a day of play together. In another section, groups of local retirees took their last sips of coffee by a warm fire as they caught up with their ski buddies and planned another fun day in the fresh air. I thought about the smiles on their faces and turned to my friend to reply. "I'm in this for the long haul. I want an activity that I can enjoy with my family as I grow older. I love the community and the way it brings people together. I love the connected feeling that I get when I ski."

MANIFEST DEEP FROM THE HEART.
DO WHAT YOU LOVE AS AN OLD FART.

Have a Vision for Health and Wellness

It was helpful to keep the endgame in mind as I continuously navigated the time pressure of getting to the mountain as often as necessary to improve. There were days when balancing my work at Nurture, managing the kids' schedules, and running the household felt as complex as overseeing a NASA mission. It was helpful to me at these times to remember the lovely 80- and

90-year-olds who sat in the lodge in the mornings, catching up over breakfast, ready to enjoy a few runs on the hill together. Watching these *masters*, I wanted to feel that same sense of ease and happiness in my elder years, that sense of connection with my body and others. I wanted to participate in this sport with my family and the broader community. When I imagined how this would feel to my 80- or 90-year-old self, it felt *good*. That is where your vision of wellness should take you.

Like Ryan, the Jedi of mindfulness, I'd also like to start you on your path to optimal wellness by first asking questions that help you to create a vision:

- What do you look like at your ideal weight and level of fitness?
- What is your ideal level of stress? Don't say none, because some level of stress is good! A stress-free life is unrealistic. We grow by challenging ourselves, and feeling a little stress can help us to be at our best. Imagine the feeling of being able to handle stress without getting overwhelmed. How does it *feel* to be in control?
- Do you have more energy and vibrancy? Where are you spending that extra energy and productivity?
- How does your physical appearance reflect your health? Are you muscular? Flexible? Able to keep up with your kids or grandkids without running out of breath?
- What does good health mean for you spiritually? Do you feel connected to something bigger than yourself?
- How are your emotions? Are you more balanced? Are you honest with yourself?

- What is the ripple effect of this vision? How are your relationships with your family, at work, and in your community affected by your good health?

Only you can answer these questions as you make your own vision of wellness. Remember to use all of your senses as you answer these questions.

The next set of questions relates to your home, and the more you can answer in the affirmative, the better.

- Is your environment clean and inspiring?
- Are you comfortable in your bed, and do you get the rest you need there?
- Do you have a place in the house where you can set up a yoga mat for a workout or a quiet retreat?
- Is your kitchen set up to inspire you to cook in a way that fits with your budget, your desires, and your time constraints?
- Do you have what you need to cook whole foods into easy dishes that you and your family love?
- Are there fresh fruits and veggies ready at hand?

THE MORE YES'S THE BETTER.
WITH A FEW NO'S, DON'T BE A FRETTER.

Resources for the No Responses

As you address your *no* responses, here are some excellent resources to consult:

- **Overall environment:** If your environment is not clean and inspiring, get Karen Kingston's book, *Clear Your Clutter with Feng Shui*. Also subscribe to the blog "Inspired Everyday Living" by sisters Alison Forbes and Laura Forbes Carlin (www.inspiredeverydayliving.com). You will feel peace and serenity in your home in no time.

- **Bedroom:** If you are not comfortable in your bed, you are not getting the sleep you need. Kingston's book and "Inspired Everyday Living" can also assist you in setting up a bedroom that is peaceful and restful. Make your bedroom setup a priority.

- **Yoga space:** If you think you do not have a place in the house where you can set up a yoga mat, I challenge you to think differently. You need a space that is only slightly larger than your mat, around 7 feet by 3 feet. For ideas on how to set up a space for home practice, read Rodney Yee's *Moving Toward Balance*.

- **Healthy eating:** The fresh-fruit-and-veggie dilemma is easy to overcome if you use your vision to plan ahead. Just remember that you are so much more likely to reach for something that is prepared rather than something that takes more work. My suggestion is that you store veggies in a grab bag when you get home from the grocery store. Wash and chop veggies and display them in containers* in your fridge within easy reach. You won't need those chips and crackers if you have something else to satisfy your oral-feedback cravings (i.e., the need to crunch on something).

---

* I always recommend BPA-free containers, especially for food storage. For BPA-free product ideas, visit www.healthysolutionsofsv.com and click on "Recommended Products" on the green navigation bar.

- **Cooking:** How can you solve the challenge of cooking whole foods into easy dishes that you and your family love? Read on. The slow cooker is coming to the rescue!

We might have solved some of your health challenges with the foundation of breakfast, but what about lunch and, especially, dinner? I've learned from many Nurture participants that the rice cooker is not the ultimate answer to the dinner dilemma because it still requires effort at the end of a long and tiring day. Daily exhaustion and dreading the preparation of dinner are exactly what send many people to the local fast food joint or down the frozen dinner route instead of making a home-cooked meal.

Nurture has a solution for those folks looking for immediate gratification as they walk through the door in the evening: a slow cooker*. This clever device allows you the flexibility to spend less than 15 minutes in the morning so that, when you get home at the end of the day, the house will smell of something delicious and inviting. The anticipation of something more nutritious and less expensive provides the willpower many of our Nurture participants need to pass up fast food restaurants on the way home from work.

As we learned from our discussion of breakfast in Mantra #2 (Get Some Good Boots On), Recipe Frameworks provide ideas for the basic components you need to prepare a meal. You can customize your choices to make a quick and easy meal

---

* For recommendations on what type of slow cooker to purchase, visit the same "Recommended Products" section; review the various slow cooker options.

based on your personal preferences and what you can find in your kitchen. You can do the same thing to prepare a dinner in your slow cooker.

Slow Cooker Recipe Framework

Meat/Protein	+	Vegetable(s)	+	Seasoning(s)	+	Liquid
turkey		carrots		garlic		water
chicken		parsnips		salt		broth
beef		leeks		pepper		olive oil
beans		onions		ginger		etc.
etc.		tomatoes		cumin		
		green onions		curry		
		frozen peas		etc.		
		etc.				

Here are some general guidelines for getting to know your slow cooker:

STEP 1:   Add ingredients according to the Recipe Framework. Always be sure there is enough liquid in the recipe so as not to burn the meal in the slow cooker.

STEP 2:   Plug in the slow cooker to a safe outlet.

STEP 3:   Cover and turn on the slow cooker.

   Guidelines are:
   • Low setting for 8-10 hours (or overnight) or high setting for 4-6 hours.

- For animal proteins, use a meat thermometer to be sure it's done.

- Turn to *keep warm* if waiting to serve.

You always can make larger quantities to freeze for the future or use leftovers for lunches or the next day's meals.

If you really like recipes, I don't want to disappoint you. For new ideas for slow cooker recipes (breakfasts, lunches, or dinners), visit the Nurture website (www.nurtureyourfamily.org) and hover over "Healthy Recipes" on the blue navigation bar. Click on "RECIPES-ADULTS" and scroll down to the section on slow cookers. You can also visit www.healthykidsideas.com and click on "Slow Cooker" under the "Search Recipes by Cooking" area on the right-hand sidebar. I doubt you will need to go further for recipe inspiration!

A SLOW COOKER IS YOUR BEST FRIEND
FOR A HOME-COOKED MEAL AT DAY'S END.

Begin with the End in Mind

When I was in management consulting in my mid and late twenties, I was more in a mode of surviving than thriving. I was climbing up the ladder of promotions, moving from consultant to senior consultant to unit manager to senior manager.

I was in no mood for relaxation, but Jeff made me take a short vacation. I threw a book into my suitcase, not realizing that it would soon change my life and my career. It was Stephen R. Covey's *The 7 Habits of Highly Effective People*. I found myself nodding in agreement through "Be Proactive" (Habit 1). Then I got to Habit 2, "Begin with the End in Mind." Covey asks the reader to picture his or her own funeral. Three people stand up to say a few words about the deceased, the type of person you were, what you stood for, how you lived, and so on. One family member, one community member, and one work colleague would speak.

"Kathryn was great with numbers and planning. She kept our family vacations on time and on budget," I heard my sister say.

"Who was Kathryn? I've only ever seen a black Audi that pulls in around midnight and leaves before dawn? Nice car," added the community member.

"Hard worker. I regularly got emails with complex attachments at 3 a.m. She sure did not need much sleep!" said a former client of mine.

Was that it? What about good daughter, sister, wife, mom? Jeff and I hadn't had any kids yet, but I always pictured myself as a mom someday. Hadn't I contributed enough to be well known—beyond a black car moving through the darkness—in my community?

Okay, I thought. I work hard, but so what?

DO WHAT YOU MUST DO.
KNOW THAT YOU CAN'T TAKE IT WITH YOU.

The Beginning of a New Ending

Over the next few years, a dramatic shift occurred in my career. We had our first child, Elena, and I continued to plug away at work, even while knowing something was off with my life balance. Then, as I was pregnant with our second child, Alexander, I was assigned to a tight-deadline project while my big belly bumped up against the desk. I had to pull two all-nighters within a week's span of time. As I was sitting at my desk wearing the same ugly maternity clothes from the previous day, I made the decision to leave the world of consulting.

"Great idea," said my mentor when I told him my news. He rubbed his hand across his smooth head. "Now that *all* of my hair is gone, I think it's time for me to leave this firm, too."

I cleaned out my office and happened to pick up my Stephen Covey book, which, by then, was sacred. What did I want my funeral to look like? What were my next steps? Needing a new mentor, I went up to South Milwaukee, Wisconsin to visit my 92-year-old grandma, who was in a retirement home. She was a beautiful, sage creature and a devout Polish Catholic. She fingered her rosary as I explained that I was at a crossroads professionally. She asked me the simplest, most profound three questions.

1. "What are your God-given gifts?"
2. "What are you passionate about?"
3. "What is a critical need in the world that is waiting to be met?"

That conversation birthed Nurture, which would grow into an important player in the national movement around nutrition and wellness education. Since I was a kid, growing up in the house of my biochemist dad, I was fascinated by the role that nutrition plays in our overall health. When my dad would take my sister and me to work, we would dive into the bookshelf to dig out the best picture books on pathology. We flipped through the pages of these medical tomes with the same engrossed attention that you see in people leafing through the *Guinness Book of World Records.*

"I can't believe this. This woman is covered with black scales and has a black tongue!"

"Eeeww! Look at this man with sores all over his body and lips!"

"Freaky. This baby has a bow-legged stance worse than an old-fashioned cowboy."

Thus I learned about pellagra, scurvy, and rickets, or, more importantly, the critical importance of such nutrients as the B, C, and D vitamins.

Thinking through my grandma's prescription, I thought:

- *God-given gifts:* Work ethic and organizational skills.
- *Passion:* Nutrition and wellness.
- *Critical need in the world:* This answer would soon be uncovered through discussions with my dad, another sage family member and mentor.

LISTEN TO WORDS OF THE WISE.
FIND YOUR PASSION, THEY ADVISE.

The Secret: Write It Down

Visualization became a big deal in the years following the 2006 release of the book and film *The Secret,* which proposes that you can be, do, have, and feel any way that you desire. Also potentially seen as woo-woo by the Wall Street types, *The Secret* is based on the law of attraction, that like attracts like. By creating our own concrete visions of how we want to live, what we want to do, what we want to have, and how we want to feel, we can actually create and influence our lives. We have the power of choice because we choose our own thoughts and our overall visions. What we think, we can attract into our lives. We can each create our own reality and our own circumstances.

When I met intuitive healer Marie Manuchehri at the 2012 Wellness Festival in Sun Valley, she talked about human beings emitting their own frequency, like a radio station. Some people tend to operate more on lower frequencies, as she described, which attract negative people, thoughts, and outcomes. With inner work, especially positive thinking and visualization, we can raise our frequency to attract more positive people, thoughts, and outcomes. In this way, we choose our future with the thoughts that we have today. What we focus on expands and affects how we feel and exerts influence on our actions. By focusing our attention on what we want to achieve, we actually transform those thought patterns into reality.

By writing down our thoughts, or representing them as images on a vision board, we give them much greater power to attract. I cannot deny that I have found this to be true in my own life.

This process transformed Nuture from an idea into a bonafide thriving organization.

On our weekly *walk and talks*, pushing the double stroller along, my dad and I took the time to catch up on life. I had just told him about an idea that had formed during my studies for my certification in nutritional counseling and my inspirational conversation with my grandmother. It was in the mid 2000s, and our walk-and-talk topics covered everything from politics to gardening to world peace. We also spent a lot of time on nutrition. My dad had been chairman of the biochemistry and anatomy departments at the Chicago Medical School. One of the courses he taught to medical students was nutrition, and he still kept up-to-date with many of the medical journals. Our conversation led from journal studies directly to the critical need in the world concept that my Grandma had mentioned.

"Have you read any of the latest statistics about Type 2 diabetes?" my dad asked.

"Yes. It is amazing how much the incidence of diabetes is increasing," I answered.

"The estimate is that one out of three children will develop diabetes if we continue to eat the standard American diet. One out of three!"

We had just stopped at a park to let my antsy kids get out and play. They were in the sandbox with a third child. I looked at them and thought: *Standard American Diet—SAD. One of those children in the sandbox would likely get diabetes!? That is sad.*

"Dad, why do you think this is happening in our country?"

"Time, money, and know-how, I suppose. People don't think they have enough money to afford good food, don't know how to prepare it, and don't feel like they have the time to help themselves. That is why fast food and processed foods are taking over."

"But, Dad, when I was in graduate school, I didn't have time or money. With my rice cooker and slow cooker, I lived off whole grains, lentils, beans, and fruits and veggies. I stayed healthy."

I recalled the parties I used to have on Wednesday nights in my 450 square foot apartment in Austin. I'd make rice and beans, and we'd gather around to watch *Melrose Place* on TV. I didn't want to admit to my dad how much fun I'd had in graduate school. His stories of living above the Bone Closet at Yale University and walking to work at his postdoc program uphill both ways through the driving snow were legends in our family. I also recall he never missed a single day of work, despite colds, high fevers, or shingles.

"Maybe I could put together a program that teaches people how to use those tools to start cooking healthy meals again," I suggested to my dad. "We could give them rice cookers and slow cookers to help them save time and make it easy to prepare healthy meals. We could focus first on low income families; they are the ones that studies show are disproportionately affected by nutritional disease."

"Write it down," my dad said.

And that vision—of a program to improve the nutrition and health of families through education—was what I wrote down. Putting the idea on paper was the best advice I could have received. Once I wrote those thoughts down, the universe started to do its part by placing people and opportunities in my path. Within a month, I had met a registered dietitian and a director of a clinical studies organization with a doctorate in nutrition, who both wanted to make the idea a reality. We called it Nurture, an acronym for Nutritional Upgrading Realized Through

Underwriting, Resources and Education. Within three months,
I had a larger group of people dedicated to making it work.
Within six months, I had start-up funds and our first program
in place with the local food pantry. I had found my calling. My
new job as the executive director of Nurture would get me out of
bed with a spring in my step for the next decade.

MANIFEST FROM HEART AND MIND.
YOUR HIGHEST CALLING YOU WILL FIND.

What Happens without Vision and Planning

There are a few very predictable phases in life. Around your late
20s and early 30s, it is common to feel that you've gone into full
wedding mode. Attending dozens of weddings a year seems normal. It was 1998 when this phase of life hit Jeff and me, and we
needed to plan for a particular wedding in Minneapolis. The
groom and dear friend of mine, John, and I met when we had
commuted from our respective parents' homes in the suburbs
for summer internships in between our sophomore and junior
years of college. John was hilarious and smart, attending Col-
gate as an English major, so I always tried to use my best SAT
words as we rode the train to work with *alacrity*. I didn't know
much about John's fiancée, Jen, except that she was very pretty
and seemed to have a great sense of humor.

I wouldn't have missed John's wedding for the world, but
Jeff and I were working on tough projects with looming dead-
lines, so we were delayed at our offices. We finally got on the

road just six hours before the wedding—with a six-hour drive ahead of us.

We arrived just in time, having driven the entire way with the top of the convertible down in the blazing sun. In our haste (and youth), we had forgotten to put on sunscreen, so when I pulled off my tank top to change into my formal strapless dress, there was a very obvious white seat belt mark in the middle of my sunburn. Our hair was standing on end, and we hadn't eaten anything since morning.

"It's a wedding," Jeff assured me. "There will be tons of food." So we sat patiently through the ceremony with our tummies grumbling as we patted down our hair. When we arrived at the reception hall, we strategically waited—like tigers perched high on the savannah—outside the door where the waiters were coming out with finger foods.

"There goes a plate of food!" I yelled as Jeff went off for an interception. He came back with a puzzled look on his face.

"Mushrooms stuffed with Spam. I didn't think you'd want one."

"Weird. Here's another waiter!" And I went in for the kill.

Spam on a stick?

This Spam surprise happened again and again as the oddest concoctions of Spam made their way by our salivating mouths. But we just couldn't get into the idea of Spam.

At dinner, we learned that Jen was somehow related to the Spam empire. On the dinner menu? Spam. And Spam.

I ate my side of carrots (with Spam) along with my champagne toast. Wow, that stuff really goes to your head when you don't have much in your system. The band started playing, and Jeff and I decided to ditch the Spam for the dance floor. Having had champagne and no food, we were less than coordinated. In fact, we were a mess. Jeff started telling me Spam jokes, and we both laughed uncontrollably and eventually fell into a room divider that was also a raised bed for plants. The entire thing crashed to the floor, dirt and flowers flying everywhere.

We were horrified. We ran.

We snuck out the back and went to the nearest place to get food at midnight in Minneapolis: Subway.

"Next time, we should really plan ahead," I said to Jeff, as we reflected on the evening.

PLAN AHEAD FOR YOUR DAY.
DON'T END UP SUNBURNED, STRIPED, SOILED,
SPAMMED, AND STARVED AT SUBWAY.

Mantra #3: Zoom out for the best view is a reminder to use vision and visualization to create the life that you want. We laymen can learn much from Olympic athletes, who spend significant time cultivating vivid, multisensory visualizations to assist them as they take on superhuman feats. When we are on the mountain skiing, we are reminded that our bodies go where we look, so it is important to know not only where to look, but also *where you want to go.* As we learned from Ryan about mindfulness, creating a vision for where our efforts will take us is a critical first step when embarking on a mind and body wellness plan. Creating a vision for wellness includes making plans ahead for meals and not waiting until the last minute. Often, our best intentions are squandered when we are faced with a hungry family at the end of a long day and there seem to be limited options. You can use the Nurture Recipe Frameworks for lunches and dinners in the slow cooker to be prepared to satisfy your family with healthy and nutritious meals. *Zoom out for the best view* is about beginning with the end in mind to avoid pushing ahead in endless activity toward an end goal that we might not understand—or want!

ACTION ITEMS FROM THIS CHAPTER

FOR SUCCESS IN LIFE:

- Pick your head up and take in the world around you. Put down your phone. Enjoy the scenery.
- Begin your projects, and life in general, with the end in mind. Determine your vision and frequently revisit it: See it, feel it, taste it—know it viscerally through your mind and your heart.
- Write your vision down to give it even more clarity and power. Let the universe help you out along the way.

FOR SUCCESS ON THE SLOPES:

- Keep your chin up. Your body goes where you are looking.
- Rely on a steady gaze to help you balance.
- Always keep in mind why you're skiing or doing any activity. Envision aging while staying active, spending time with your spouse and family, or whatever long-term benefits you associate with the outdoors and exercise.

FOR SUCCESS IN WELLNESS:

- Create a vision of what it feels like to be healthy. Understand how this vision would affect you personally as well as others around you. Reflect daily on that impact, especially in the morning and as you go to bed, and the motivation to make change will arise naturally.
- Create a gap between a stimulus and your response to enable you to make a choice that helps you reach your goals.
- Plan your meals ahead and involve your inner artist in cooking by using the Recipe Frameworks for the slow cooker.

Mantra #4
Plant Your Poles

We need a balance between lazy and crazy.

KYLE CEASE

2014 and 2015 Sun Valley Wellness Festival speaker

Taking in an expansive view from a mountaintop is one thing, but being able to descend from the top safely is another thing entirely. Setting a vision for what we want to achieve in life is a great start, but we must be able to take the vision into mind and then create actionable, measurable steps that we feel are attainable. A vision—whether it's for work, wellness, or life overall—can often be so overwhelming that it prevents us from moving forward. It's easy to face the same problem when looking at a long, challenging ski run in its entirety; it seems like simply too much to handle. I've learned that breaking down a ski run into a series of manageable turns—each with its own *pole plant*—is the way to overcome the fear of starting the journey. Pole planting describes how skiers use poles when executing turns. To maintain speed and control, it's important to firmly put the tip of your pole into the snow on the inside of a turn. This gives you a pivot point to work from as you change direction.

Bust through Boundaries

It was the 2013–14 winter season, and I was manifesting a mountain life from my heart and mind. I was planning to ski into my old age alongside Jeff and my kids. We would have time to play as a family outdoors and stay connected, balanced, and healthy. The only thing that seemed to be a problem with achieving my vision was that my family loved to spend time exploring the bumps and near the trees. Skiers refer to this area as "off the groomers" because it is the part of a mountain that isn't groomed by large machines designed to maintain recreational trails. I hadn't ventured off the groomers yet, so I couldn't go with them, and I was unsure of to how to move forward. Then, I heard a wonderful story from one of my Nordic ski coaches, a two-time U.S. Olympian, Betsy Youngman—and it helped me gain the courage to try new terrain.

"I told myself to explore what lay beyond the flags, just a little at a time," Betsy explained to me as I soaked up her knowledge and experience. She wasn't talking about flags along a ski run. I was interviewing her about her six-week stay at a research station on the ice cap of Greenland, where she was part of a team conducting climate studies.

"On the ice cap in Greenland, everything is white at times, up and down and right and left. In these conditions, it is extremely easy to become disoriented," she said. "So the base station had put up flags around the area in the snow where we were supposed to stay when we ventured away from the safety of camp. When I would go out for my morning ski on the crust, I began to ache to go explore beyond those flags."

I sympathized with her. A woman who can ski a dazzling 20 kilometers an hour and radiates energy even while standing still, she must have felt like a fish in a tiny bowl as she did her morning laps.

"The flags became a metaphor for boundaries in life, kind of like a horizon that you can't see beyond. I knew that, while I didn't want to risk endangering myself, I did want to explore just a little more. I wanted to go just beyond the flags, a very small amount at a time."

"I didn't know what lay beyond the flags. But like any horizon line, my curiosity drove me towards the edge," Betsy continued, smiling and speaking words of a very wise Olympic rock star.

INCREMENTAL PROGRESS IN AN EXPANSE OF WHITE
IS THE WAY TO FIND GREATER DELIGHT.

Set Goals with Your Poles

Intellectually, I could understand that setting goals is about taking a big vision and breaking it down into manageable chunks. But this idea of manageable pieces was a tough one to conjure when I was standing above a double-black diamond bump run, appropriately named Rock Garden. It looked like a vast sea of egg cartons, all turned upside down, creating a massive network of moguls through which we would need to make our way.

"Set your intention," urged Davina, the day's energetic instructor. "The pole plant before your turn is always important. In the moguls, it is essential. When you ski through the moguls, you are setting a series of intentions with each pole plant. And keep in mind that each intention comes quickly!"

We went through our drill, saying the word *intention* as we planted our pole before each turn. The pole plant was a reach forward and down in the direction that we wanted to go, but it wasn't so far ahead that we were stretching our arms. It was just far enough to get us from one turn, and one mogul, to the next.

The pole plant became my metaphor for setting goals as I started to explore terrain off the groomed runs. A huge line of bumps seemed overwhelming and scary, when taken as a whole, in the same way that a vision for what you want to accomplish in life might be overwhelming if you look at it as too large a picture. I realized how important it is to take that vision and break it down into manageable steps. These steps become your goals. Thinking about the process this way, the long and steep bump run was now just a series of intentions and pole plants and, therefore, quite achievable after all. This realization was a huge turning point in my skiing, in part because moguls opened up so much new terrain for me. Moreover, in life, my realization also allowed me to see how a vision can be broken down into smaller, manageable steps.

BUMP BY BUMP, DOWN THE LINE
IS THE WAY TO FEEL SAFE AND FINE.

Don't Be a Herbie

As I was making progress with alpine skiing (often referred to as *downhill skiing*) through DIVAS, I learned about a local women's group for Nordic, or *cross-country,* skiing, called VAMPS (short for Vimin And Muffy's Programs). Our sunny ski town sure had a thing for catchy acronyms. Muffy is the legendary Muffy Ritz. To explain why I call her legendary, I will start with the true story about her winning the grueling 55-kilometer Birkebeiner cross-country race in Wisconsin—*the first time she put on Nordic skis.* I had heard locals talking about how much they loved being part of VAMPS, as long as you were up for a suffer fest.

I didn't know Muffy, but I had seen her around our neighborhood a few miles north of town center. One afternoon, we were driving home from the grocery store in a huge winter storm, winds blowing fiercely as the snow piled in drifts.

"Hey, Mom, do you see that really strong lady on the bike? She has her groceries, too. Except she biked to the store, unlike us," Alexander said in admiration and awe of Muffy. "And she is being a good steward of the environment," chimed in Elena, who was counting carbon imprint points for her school environmental project. Our car trip to the store had just cost her dearly.

"I saw her doing some push-ups and pull-ups at the park," Alexander added. "You should just try to keep up with her."

When I joined VAMPS, that same winter season, I had a vision that I could do the famous, or perhaps infamous, Boulder Tour with the team. Muffy let me join VAMPS once I assured her I had completed the Sun Valley Half Marathon successfully. She doesn't allow rank beginners in the group because they slow everyone down, as I would learn all too soon.

Back in graduate school, as part of the operations-management curriculum, I read *The Goal,* a short but powerful book co-authored by Dr. Eliyahu M. Goldratt, an Israeli physicist, educator, and business leader. The most memorable concept of the book is the *Herbie*, a single element that slows down the entire production process. In the book, Herbie is a pudgy and slow Boy Scout on a hike with the rest of his fit and fast group. Herbie's lack of fitness becomes a problem for the entire group because they need to stick together.

The point is that we need to keep our eyes out for the Herbies of the world because, by speeding them up, we can speed up entire systems.

"You are an AmeriCAN, not an AmeriCAN'T!" Muffy encouraged us as we did another lap around the Nordic training circuit. We were testing speed levels for groups that would ski the Boulder Tour together. The Boulder Tour is a 33-kilometer, one-way Nordic course. The logistics require that you leave a car at the finish line, drive a second car to the starting point, and then, once everyone has finished, drive back to retrieve the other vehicle. In other words, the course requires that you stick together as a group. Since I was finishing my laps nearly 30 minutes after the others, I knew I would be a drag on everyone. People would freeze as they waited for me before retrieving the second car. Even though the Boulder Tour had been my vision when I started Nordic skiing, I was now having trouble realizing it.

"Don't fret it," Muffy said. "You just need to break it down. Don't start with a 33K course but a 5K one, instead. Build your technique on that distance. Then build your endurance. Keep increasing your distance until you're ready. The Boulder Tour will be waiting for you later."

Breaking down my vision into manageable goals turned out to be a win-win-win for my team, my coaches, and me that first year of VAMPS. Alongside my DIVAS Best Attitude Award sits my other most-cherished award, the Coach's Award, given to the VAMPS member deemed most coachable for that year. My willingness to set realistic, attainable goals that pushed me brought success to my team. For the record, the next season I finished the Boulder Tour with Team Guylay: Jeff, Elena, Alexander, and me.

**TAKE ONE RACE AT A TIME.
DON'T SLOW DOWN THE ENTIRE LINE.**

Put the Horse before the Cart

I appreciated that Muffy was willing to be patient and break down a long, challenging process into a series of steps. That is what goal setting is all about, and I had experienced this discipline when managing client expectations through long consulting processes.

"Show me the money!" a sales manager said to me at our first project meeting.

"Excuse me?" I asked.

"Haven't you ever seen the movie *Jerry Maguire*? Show me the money!"

The client, a technology products company, had engaged our consulting firm to design an incentive plan for the sales organization, which had failed to meet its financial targets over the past five years.

The CEO had invited the sales manager to our first project meeting, and I got the impression that he was eager for immediate change. He seemed to believe that the incentive plan was flawed, so it didn't properly reward him and his team. My guess was that the plan didn't offer adequate financial awards to top salespeople, but I wasn't sure, and I knew we couldn't fix the situation then and there.

"I can't design a new sales incentive plan solution right here and now," I told him.

"Why not?"

"A sales incentive plan is a tool to direct people to execute a strategy."

"Strategy?"

Then a pause. "A strategy is a plan of action to achieve a set of goals. Goals that ultimately lead to a common vision," I offered.

"Vision?" stammered the sales manager. Another pause.

"I can't give you a sales incentive plan solution without a clear understanding of what your company's visions and goals are. I can't put the cart before the horse. The vision, goals, and strategy need to come first. Then, the sales incentive plan will follow."

I turned to the CEO, and we proceeded to outline a series of executive interviews to establish a common vision. We would then set goals that led toward that vision. Goals would be five-year, one-year, six-month and, finally, monthly. Goals would be meaningful yet attainable. We would know who was responsible for doing what and when. This action plan was our strategy: a step-by-step outline mapping out how goals would be achieved.

With a vision, goals, and a strategy in place, designing a great incentive plan was straightforward. And the sales team made its revenue and profit targets for the first time in five years. How? Because the incentive plan aligned perfectly with the organization's overall strategy and clearly directed what everyone needed to do. We put the horse before the cart.

STEP-BY-STEP, PUT THINGS IN ORDER.
AVOID A CART-AND-HORSE DISORDER.

Focus and the Sausage Factory

It's not that putting together a successful sales incentive plan for that technology company was easy. It took more than four months and required that we constantly check in with the answers to questions such as, "Why are we doing all of this work in the first place?" Breaking down the overall process into manageable pieces, much like breaking down a long mogul run into a series of manageable turns, requires focus. Focus requires that we check in with our brain and, from time to time, quiet the noise in there.

Our brain processes many thoughts, kind of like a sausage factory sending out link after link after link, all day long. The average person has thousands of thoughts per day; the exact number is disputed, ranging from 2,000 up to 70,000. The point is that we have many, and our thoughts play a major role in shaping how each day goes.

I think about the hikes I took when we first moved to Sun Valley. The scenery was beautiful, but the views competed with a huge, ongoing dialogue inside my head.

That was an interesting juicing class the other day. I really should go pick up some greens at the store and try some of the recipes.

What was the name of that book again? I wanted to pick it up after the class but I forgot.

Didn't my sister Suzanne say she was interested in juicing? When is the last time I talked to her? I should call her.

I have a bunch of phone calls I need to make. Ooops. I forgot to call back the orthodontist. I needed to change Elena's appointment because we are going to be away next month visiting Chicago.

We are leaving soon! I need to set up the dog-sitter! I'll ask her to water our plants, too.

What about all the edible plants that I wanted to start before the season gets too hot? I should call the garden store and get some advice on how to catch up on the gardening season.

And on and on and on. My brain was constantly being hijacked.

Is this normal? In *S.C.O.R.E. for Life*, Jim Fannin, the coach of top athletes, proposes that true champions have far fewer thoughts than non-champions. He describes the thoughts of the non-champion as bouncing around like a pinball, shifting from the past to the future and back again in just seconds. Entering the mind of a champion, one finds peace and focus in the present moment. Fannin calls that state "The Zone" and believes it is the key to success in sports, business, and life. The Zone is not a place of multi-tasking and ruminating; it's one of focus.

Fannin's theory rang true to me, so I set out to quiet my mind.

Ha! Easier said than done.

I went to my first guided meditation retreat. Many yoga and mindfulness classes later, I stumbled upon a book that, at first glance, had nothing to do with mindfulness. It was David Allen's *Getting Things Done*, a book created for people who want to be more productive and efficient. A major takeaway from Allen's book is that you must get all of your to-do's into a documented system that you trust; then you can actually allow your mind to be empty. What a concept! Rather than forcing my mind to be quiet while it struggled to remind me of my to-do list, this book suggested an alternative way of getting to the same state. Get your list out of your memory, write it down somewhere else, and trust that it will get done.

After reading his book, I cleaned up my email and physical desk based on the action folders of Allen's system and started to feel calm at work again. When out for a hike or ski, I let my mind rest and be free from the to-do's. As a result of this mind space, I started to feel more creative. If something popped into my head to distract me from the present moment, I used the Voice Memos app on my phone to record it and then cleared my mind again. What I noticed was that if I trusted that I would get to everything via the systems I had in place, I could allow myself to be fully present in each moment, with a silent, rather than chattering, mind. If I went to a meeting, I listened fully. If I was making dinner, I was truly engrossed in the smells and textures of the food I was preparing. If I went into the mountains, I would smell the air, see the contrasting colors, and enjoy myself. My productivity skyrocketed along with my creativity. I realized that the human mind is much like a computer, with an amazing ability to keep multiple programs up and running at the same time, if we request. But there is a huge cost to switching back and forth between programs,

ranging from simply slowing down the system overall to actually crashing and losing your data.

MAKE THE MIND QUIET.
AVOID A SAUSAGE-FACTORY RIOT.

Your Mind as a Garden

Was it possible to think less and produce more? I learned the
answer to this question as I tended my small but precious edible garden. I have received great advice from my professional
gardening friends, Jeanne Nolan and Chrissie Huss. Consistently, I hear from them:

"Kathryn, you need to *thin* your plants!"

The dreaded thinning process means pulling out or cutting
back perfectly healthy seedlings that have come up too close to
their neighbor plants. Tight spacing is a side effect of my method of seeding, which is to sprinkle the seeds into the dirt rather
than to count out the recommended number per square foot. I
know that not every seed will germinate, so I like to think I'm
reducing the risk of a bare garden, but my seedlings are often
too numerous for their space.

I gaze over my crowded garden boxes with sadness.

Only 16 carrot seedlings per square foot? Only four rainbow
chard plants? Only one tomato plant?!

How painful to kill perfectly healthy plants that are beneficial and could feed my family.

Wah! Wah! Wah! I think as the thinning sheers of death
hover above these beautiful baby plants.

Experienced gardeners like Jeanne and Chrissie know that thinning is ultimately beneficial and yields more productivity. When I refrain from thinning, my plants aren't tall and robust, root vegetables never grow, and my time is ultimately wasted. While it may be painful, thinning is necessary.

Our minds are similar to gardens in that some openness and space are actually required for our most productive thoughts to grow and flourish. I have resisted this idea in the past, thinking that *clearing the mind* was just an excuse to not apply yourself.

Dan Harris asked, when he wrote his book on meditation, *10% Happier*, "If I quiet the voice in my head, will I lose my edge?" The answer, Harris found, as supported by many other studies on meditation, is that you don't need "compulsive worry" to be successful. Quite to the contrary, quieting the mind allows you to tap into your potential for creativity. As Feng Shui urges you to de-clutter, jettison the old papers from your drawers and clothes from your closet so you can bring in the new, meditation aims to get the clutter out of your head to allow fresh and new thoughts to take root and expand.

The metaphor of the mind as a garden also helps us to understand the detrimental nature of negative thoughts. Negative thoughts are the mind's weeds. They will not only crowd out your genius, but also consume space and resources and leave you with nothing beneficial. You may not be able to get rid of all negative thoughts, but be on the constant lookout for how many weeds are sprouting and why.

MAKE GARDEN AND MIND WEED-FREE.
MAXIMIZE FREEDOM AND CREATIVITY.

Life Is Long

Say you've set your vision, you have goals, and you're getting focused. You've weeded out negativity and feel like you're ready to skyrocket ahead. If you're like me, you then want to get everything done *now*. But this moment might instead be the perfect time to simply take a deep breath and wait.

While visiting with my mother-in-law, Terry, I asked her advice regarding my next steps with Nurture. After the initial start-up of the organization, we experienced rapid growth and a need to add positions and systems. There was a lot of work to do, and I wanted to bite off huge chunks at once. Her words stopped me in my tracks.

"Slow down. Life is long."

She reminded me that I had two small children at home. She herself had stayed home for 15 years to raise her kids before going back to school to get her CPA and MBA. She then rose through the ranks of an accounting firm and landed the job of her dreams in an investment management company in her 50s. She was now in her 60s and felt that she had accomplished everything that she had set out to do professionally.

As Aaron Hurst says in his book, *The Purpose Economy*, "Most of us will work for 45 to 50 years. Think about that for a second. That is the same amount of time it would take to attend college twelve times ... During that time, we will hold many different jobs ... in a range of fields! We have so many opportunities to find the work that best suits our perspective on the world and the way we most enjoy contributing."

"Don't rush things," Terry urged. "You will have time to get done what you need to do, even if it doesn't always seem that way."

We happened to be having this conversation while driving down the road in Port Washington, New York, where a scene from the movie *Meet the Parents* was filmed. Ben Stiller's character was racing Robert De Niro's character to get back to the house to check on a lost cat, Jinxy. Each character would floor the gas pedal and rapidly speed to the next stoplight, which would comically turn red just as their cars arrived, forcing them to screech to a halt. They glared at each other intently until the light turned green. Then, they would speed off to the next red light, only to wait again with increased anxiety. I noticed that a lot of drivers in New York have a tendency to hurry up and wait. Drivers would speed by us, recklessly changing lanes while giving us the finger for driving at the speed limit. But we inevitably saw those same cars and those same people at the next red light. I looked over at the extremely anxious and impatient drivers at the stoplight and tried not to laugh.

I agreed with Terry right then and there that I couldn't rush things. I would set my vision and direct my actions proactively with goals, but I wouldn't be a jerk about making things happen on a forced timeline.

GO WITH THE FLOW OF LIFE'S PACE.
DON'T GET IN A STOP-AND-GO DRAG RACE.

Balance Receptivity with Proactivity

Journalist Jen Weigel suggests a practice of balancing proactivity with receptivity. She starts each day by doing three to five action-oriented steps (e.g., making an outreach call, sending an article to her editor, completing an interview) that will set events in motion. She then steps back and consciously allows receptivity to take over.

Jen explains, "The universe is like a cargo plane that wants to make a delivery to you when you've asked for help, but it looks for a landing strip that is free of debris. It is looking for a safe and quiet place to deliver you its goods. If your landing strip happens to have geese and people running this way and that in general chaos, the cargo plane will look for somewhere else more peaceful to land. It always will prefer an open field that is quiet and serene. To receive from the universe, you either need to clean up your own landing strip or be that quiet and calm field."

For those of us who have learned to succeed in life by trying to force a plane to land in chaos, it is time to soften the approach. As yoga instructor Baron Baptiste says in his book, *Journey Into Power,* "Trying hard invites strain and struggle. Trying easy gives you the levity and freedom to fly."

TRY EASY WITHOUT UNDUE STRESS;
IT'S THE WAY TO GREATER SUCCESS.

Wellness Goals Don't Have to Be Dull

Every year in January, when the overindulgences of the holiday season pass, people sign up in droves for gyms and make resolutions to be healthy once and for all. The sad truth about these New Year's resolutions is that the majority of them fail because people's default position in life is to take the easiest route or, at least, the most fun one. Because of this basic human tendency, I urge you to make your health goals actionable and fun. Act like a kid again. You might be getting tired of my rhymes by now, but I can't seem to help myself in wanting to help you set fun goals. I might not be the best, but I'm on a quest! Here are some goals that I urge you to adopt on your way to better eating:

- Shun portion distortion
- Celebrate MyPlate
- Follow the rainbow
- Rethink your drink

Shun Portion Distortion

"Table for two," Valla, a friend of mine, said with a bit of disgust as he, Jeff, and I walked into a seafood restaurant in the heart of downtown Chicago. It was a busy night. The hostess looked at our group of *three* with suspicion.

"Just *ugh*. These guys are newlyweds. They can sit on each other's laps."

"Excuse me?" said the hostess.

"It's ridiculous. When they speak to each other all I hear is 'smootchy whooshey,'" Valla continued. "It's really annoying. But trust me, they'll share a chair. And probably a meal, too."

The hostess was still looking at him with confusion. Valla was a medical student doing one of his rotations at a Chicago hospital. Rather than get his own apartment for his short three months in town, he had asked if he could stay in our living room on Lake Shore Drive. "Of course, Dr. Valla," we told him. "Just as long as you don't mind being the third wheel." Valla knew us well enough to know what he was getting into.

The hostess led us to a table in the corner.

"Seriously," Valla said to her. "Just count them as one person. They will certainly eat off the same plate."

That was indeed true. Jeff and I loved to go out to dinner every Friday night, but we had learned over time that eating an entire entrée each was simply too much, so we always picked one to share.

It was my turn to order. "We'll have the herb crusted ..."

"Salmon, please," finished Jeff. I smiled at him in agreement.

As much as our finishing each other's sentences annoyed Valla, he conceded the point that restaurant portions had ballooned way out of control. He had heard a story about how the Center for Science in the Public Interest had recently started including a section in its newsletter called "Food Porn."

"Finally, we doctors are starting to pay attention," said Valla, as he smiled and eyed the table of six women next to us on a girls' night out.

"Food porn! What does *that* mean?" I said too loudly.

"They are comparing what the food industry is doing, like how some companies are creating packaging for snacking in reasonable portions. Then, on the same page, they show some really outrageous stuff. They call that the *food porn*."

At the mention of porn, several of the girls at the nearby table looked over. Valla was really good-looking, the tall, dark, and mysterious type.

"Can you give me an example of food porn?" asked Jeff, interrupting Valla's stare at the other table.

"The magazine article picks out a food item or entrée that goes beyond the limits of acceptable societal norms," Valla said. "Having 2,000 calories per serving, three days' worth of saturated fat, or a week's worth of sodium. It's fascinating, yet a bit disgusting at the same time."

Our food arrived, and we were about to settle in. Jeff and I decided to share a fork.

"You know what, guys? I'm outta here," Valla said.

Then, to the many giggles of the table beside us, Valla abandoned us and joined the girls-night-out-table. We didn't see him until the next day.

SHARING AT RESTAURANTS IS MY ADVICE, NOT TO BE NAUGHTY BUT TO BE NICE.

Portion Distortion Over Time

Several generations ago, it might not have been as critical for us to follow a rule such as splitting an entrée when dining out. Portion distortion is a relatively new phenomenon in the food industry, and it is critical for your health that you understand the implications of the changes in portion size over time.

When McDonald's first opened in 1955, it offered one drink size: 6.5 ounces. Today, the kids' size is 12 ounces, and the large is 32 ounces! As you may know, choosing soda as a beverage is not an optimal choice, but what if you do decide to have a soda once in a while? What are the implications of having one of today's large sodas as compared to 1955's 6.5-ounce serving?

The difference is an extra 245 calories and 17.5 teaspoons of sugar! To burn the extra calories in a single large soda would take nearly an hour of biking.

Michael Bloomberg, the former mayor of New York City, didn't think all the soda drinkers out there would burn the additional calories with physical activity. Concerned about the growing costs of diabetes and other nutrition-related diseases, he proposed limits on the sale of sugary drinks in an effort to keep servings to 16 ounces or less. Unfortunately, his proposal was overturned.

What about bagels? In the past 40 years, bagels have nearly doubled in size. The three-inch diameter bagels that I remember as a kid had about 140 calories, much fewer than the 350 calories in the six-inch bagels you often find at stores today.

The calorie difference between the bagel of the 1970s and a bagel of today is about 210 calories, and most of that comes from processed grains that will turn from sugar to fat in your body unless you burn it off first. In other words, you'd better be running those two miles to the bagel shop—assuming you want to stay as svelte as those '70s disco stars.

**MAKE SURE TO RUN TO THAT DELI
TO AVOID A BAGEL AROUND YOUR BELLY.**

Serving Size Does Not Equal Portion Size

A critical first step is to understand the difference between a *serving size* and a *portion size*. A serving size is a specified amount shown on the Nutrition Facts label on a package. The information there, including the number of calories, applies to the serving size. A portion is how much you actually eat or drink in one sitting; it is also the amount of food you get in a single restaurant order. Guess what: On average, one portion size is equal to two or three serving sizes. Food packaging is tricky, and most people don't do the math to realize how many calories they are actually consuming. Shoppers might see 250 calories per serving on the Nutrition Facts label but end up eating the entire box or bag in one sitting. They forget to multiply the number of calories by the number of servings. If there are two servings in the package, they've just eaten 500 calories, not 250. When reading a Nutrition Facts label, before you read any of the other information, always start by looking at the number of servings.

Once you know the difference between the amount of food in a serving and the amount in a portion, you can use strategies to control the size of your portions. We've already discussed sharing an entrée at a restaurant. If you don't have anyone to share with, simply ask your waiter to save half of your entrée in a to-go bag and have it for lunch the following day. At home, use a 9-inch plate instead of a 12-inch plate. The visual cue of a full plate, even one that's smaller, can lead to satisfaction. Don't eat directly from the box or bag. Pour a serving onto a plate and put the container away. Finally, use a comparison to everyday objects to get a sense of what a reasonable portion size is. I have never weighed my food, nor do I count grams or calories on a daily basis. I control my portions by understanding what is a reasonable amount of food to add to my plate. Here are the guidelines I follow:

- Carbohydrates. Amount: ½ cup cooked, about the size of half a baseball.
- Protein. Amount: 3 ounces, about the size of a deck of cards.
- Dairy. Amount: 1 ounce, about the size of four dice.
- Nut butter. Amount: 1 tablespoon, about the size of half a ping-pong ball.
- Oils and dressings. Amount: 2 tablespoons, about the size of one ping-pong ball.
- Vegetables. Amount: Unlimited, pile them up without worrying about quantities!

SIZE FOOD AS A BALL OR CARD DECK TO KEEP PORTION SIZES IN CHECK.

Celebrate MyPlate

I have been in the nutrition education field long enough to consider myself a survivor of the *plague of the pyramids*. If you do not remember the original diabetes-inducing diagram from the 1990s, which led people to eat bread by the loaf, consider yourself lucky. Thank goodness for Michelle Obama and her efforts to create a healthy and easy-to-understand visual aid to illustrate nutritional guidelines*.

MyPlate is a nutritional icon that I'm happy to use as a teaching tool. It can help you turn your vision for wellness into a reality

---

* See www.choosemyplate.gov for more information about MyPlate

because you can use it to set goals. Here are the key take-aways that Nurture teaches with MyPlate:

- Make half of your plate fruits and veggies, with an emphasis on the veggies!
- Eat lean protein. My dad's rule for breakfast applies to every snack and meal throughout the day.
- Make your grains whole grains. While MyPlate asks for only half your grains to be whole, I recommend avoiding processed grains whenever possible.
- Choose your beverage wisely. You know the saying "You are what you eat," but our diabetes issues nationally are also very much related to what we drink. Cut out the soda and sugary drinks. Kids should not have more than one cup of fruit juice a day (or better yet, none). And no large sodas, please.

Another plate-based nutritional teaching tool that I love is Harvard's Healthy Eating Plate*. This adaptation of MyPlate highlights water, not dairy, as the beverage of choice. I also appreciate the addition of the healthy oils on the side. There are a few other differences as well, but both are far better than the disastrous food pyramid.

CHOOSE HARVARD'S HEALTHY OR MYPLATE FOR ADVICE THAT MAKES YOU FEEL GREAT.

---

* See www.health.harvard.edu/healthy-eating-plate for more information about Harvard's Healthy Eating Plate.

Follow the Rainbow

When interviewing Olympic athletes about their eating practices, I expected to hear complex methods and formulas, given that each athlete generally works with a specialized sports nutritionist. The reality is that Olympians apply concepts that are simple enough for everyone to follow. One of these guidelines is to *eat the rainbow* when choosing fruits and veggies. In fact, the U.S. Ski Team often adds competitive flair to their mealtimes by seeing who can create the most colorful plate when visiting the salad bar. The minimum goal is to get three colors, but the more the healthier!

Foods' natural colors often correlate to certain micronutrients. For example, red is associated with lycopene and heart health. Orange and yellow fruits and vegetables often are loaded with vitamin A, which supports your immune system as well as skin and vision health. Green is associated with folate and other B-vitamins as well as calcium, which is good for your bones and teeth and the digestive and cardiovascular systems. The blue and purple group will assure you a bounty of antioxidants, which support healthy aging. White is associated with potassium and fiber, found in veggies such as jicama, potatoes, and mushrooms. When you go to the grocery store, challenge yourself (and your kids!) to find different fruits and veggies in various colors. (Note: When it comes to eating a rainbow, Skittles obviously do not count.)

EAT COLORS FROM NATURE OR FARMS,
NOT DIAMONDS AND CLOVERS FROM LUCKY CHARMS.

Rethink Your Drink

Our country is on a sugar-driven runaway train headed for disaster, and sugary drinks are greasing the rails. The average teenager consumes an estimated 34 teaspoons of added sugar every single day. Sugar consumption is linked to such maladies as tooth decay, obesity, Type 2 diabetes, a suppressed immune system, and stunted growth due to too little vitamin and mineral intake. When Nurture teaches kids about beverages, we first start by reminding them that we all need to drink enough liquids to stay hydrated. Dehydration causes headaches, hunger, upset stomach, crabbiness, fatigue, and difficulty concentrating. Our bodies are comprised of more than 60 percent water; proper hydration regulates body temperature, transports nutrients to our cells, and protects organs and tissues. Water also removes waste. Staying hydrated is one of the most important things we can do for our health.

Once we've convinced the students how important it is to drink enough fluids, we move on to reviewing options. We compare beverage choices and ask students to give each one a prize. Just like the Olympics, we have bronze, silver, and gold medals.

First, we look at soda. We see that soda provides no nutritional value. It is loaded with sugar and sometimes caffeine. It is estimated that the average American consumes 592 cans of soda per year —and the 32-plus pounds of sugar that go with it! While diet sodas don't contain sugar, they also provide no nutritional value and contain many artificial ingredients that can be harmful to bodies and brains. It is best to limit soda to a *sometimes* or, better yet, *never* beverage. Soda doesn't get any medal at all.

Sports and energy drinks don't make it to the podium either. Many people think that sports drinks are healthy, but they contain a lot of sugar, artificial ingredients, and dyes. The electrolytes found in sports drinks are only needed when people are being so active that they sweat for an hour or more. If your kids need to replace electrolytes, then I recommend drinking water and taking an electrolyte replacement tablet*. That way, they can stay hydrated and replenish their electrolytes without the artificial ingredients, sugars, and dyes found in sports drinks. You can also offer your kids water with a squeeze of fruit or veggie juice and maybe a pinch of salt, if they've really had a sweat fest. All fruits and veggies provide potassium, a key electrolyte; bananas are standouts when it comes to this mineral, and coconut water is an even better source.

When we get to fruit juice, we are now on the podium, but juice only comes in as the bronze medal winner of what we call the *better beverages*. Real, 100 percent juice contains vitamins and minerals but also a lot of natural sugar. Keep an eye out for juice look-alikes that are not 100 percent juice. Look past the marketing and read the ingredient list to make sure the drink is not a fruit or veggie wannabe.

Milk (but not chocolate milk) is our silver-medal winner for better beverages. Milk contains calcium and vitamin D, which help build strong bones and teeth. Not everyone tolerates milk well, so kids should listen to their bodies and tummies to make sure that milk agrees with them.

---

* For electrolyte tablets/capsules, visit www.healthysolutionsofsv.com and click on "Recommended Products" on the green navigation bar.

The gold medal goes to water! Water gives you a long-lasting hydration boost and contains no sugar, dyes, or artificial ingredients. The best part about water is that it is usually available and free. If students realize that water is the number-one choice but still want something special to dazzle the taste buds, I recommend *wuice*. Wuice is water with a little bit of juice added from any fruit or veggie. For a flavorful refresher, add cucumber rounds, citrus slices, watermelon cubes, or berries.

WHEN THIRSTY, REACH FOR H_2O, THE GOLD MEDAL WAY TO GO.

All Is Fine with a Rhyme

Everyone has personal techniques to relieve stress and find a little humor in life. I like to rhyme, which you've certainly figured out by now. Here are a few more, dripping with cheese (if you please).

- Eat breakfast every day, be energized for work and play.
- Eat protein with every meal, see how great you feel.
- For grains, choose whole, and practice quality control.
- Fruits and veggies fill your plate, for a healthy body weight.

If you have kids at home, rhyming can be a way to keep conversations about food fun and positive. For great messaging about eating colorful fruits and vegetables, I recommend the book *Give It a Go, Eat a Rainbow* (to be published in 2016 by

Kathryn Kemp Guylay and award-winning food photographer
Paulette Phlipot), which includes an engaging rhyme story ac-
companied by beautiful artistic images.

KEEP IT POSITIVE AND FUN
FOR GOOD HEALTH IN THE LONG RUN.

Mantra #4: Plant your poles is a reminder that we must
break down our expansive vision into realistic and achievable
steps. In skiing, we set a goal every single time we plant our
poles. Off the mountain, we can plant our metaphorical poles to
establish the direction we want to go and to set an intention for
what comes next. I encourage you to set intentions whenever
you embark on a new project or journey. As Muffy taught us, we
do ourselves a disservice if we try to tackle the entire course at
once. We need to challenge ourselves in work, life, and health,
but we must also have a sense of how we can achieve the goals
we set. We should have patience along the way instead of trying
to force outcomes. Life is long. We should endeavor to quiet our
minds, removing negative thoughts like pulling weeds from a
garden. We should wrangle complex topics into a system that is
not only actionable but also fun. *Plant your poles* is about turning your vision into reality, one turn at a time.

ACTION ITEMS FROM THIS CHAPTER

FOR SUCCESS IN LIFE:

- Break down your goals into manageable pieces. Life is long and should not be rushed.
- Focus. Quiet your mind to allow for greater productivity and creativity.
- Balance proactivity and receptivity. Don't always try hard, try easy.

FOR SUCCESS ON THE SLOPES:

- Don't start with a double black diamond or a 33K Nordic race, even if that is your vision. Break your vision down into manageable goals that you can achieve season by season and day by day.
- Know that even if you don't know what's next, it's fun to explore if you take it in small steps.
- Be ambitious and realistic with your abilities. Ultimately, you will go far, even if it doesn't feel that way at every moment.

FOR SUCCESS IN WELLNESS:

- With a vision of your own wellness in mind, create goals that are actionable, achievable, and measurable.
- Start your list of health goals with the following memorable rhymes: 1) shun portion distortion, 2) celebrate MyPlate, 3) follow the rainbow, and 4) rethink your drink.
- When possible, make your health goals positive rather than punitive. Enjoy the journey.

Embrace the Yard Sale

Everything serves.

—DR. SUE MORTER
international speaker and master of bioenergetic medicine

In skiing slang, you have a yard sale when you fall down and lose all your equipment—skis pop off, poles get lost, and snow gets into every last crevice of your being. Most skiers experience yard sales from time to time; at least one advantage of falling on snow is that it typically provides a nice, soft landing. Falling, only to get up and start again, is one of the key elements of skiing and, like failing, it is one of the most important ways humans learn. We get so caught up in the notions of success and perfection that we often forget to acknowledge and appreciate failure. One of the most important things I've learned through spending time in the mountains is that there is no such thing as perfection. Let go of the crazy, high standards you might have for yourself and start learning to appreciate failure. Another thing I have learned from skiing is that strength and balance come from the core, not from our extremities. When I fall and fail in life, I notice that I have often strayed from the strength of my core. When I succeed, I know that I am gathering power from my center and am on the right path.

Cod Liver Oil

"Kathryn, you need to join us on our weekend suffer fests," Muffy Ritz, head of the VAMPS women's Nordic program, said happily.

I had just finished my first Nordic practice race, and coming in last place had not helped my overall sense of well-being or confidence. I was also not feeling the best in terms of tummy comfort.

Muffy continued, "You need to accept a little failure and learn from what you are doing wrong. How about you join our group on the weekends when we do sprints? They are not fun, but they are short, improve your speed, and amplify the areas where you need work. *Cod liver oil*, we call them."

Cod liver oil? It sounded awful, but what was I going to say? I was talking to one of my skiing idols.

"Okay. I'll give it a try. See you next weekend," I said, as I limped away.

I showed up the following weekend for the practice races and quickly learned why they're affectionately called cod liver oil. The drills were fast circuits, often with grueling uphill stretches that made my lungs burn and my legs scream for mercy. We practiced short sprints, which I find much more difficult than the longer circuits, in which the trick is simply to pace yourself. The exertion triggered both fight and flight responses in me, as the reptilian part of my brain fixated on the sign at the end of the circuit that said, "FINISHING IS YOUR ONLY EFFING OPTION." My race was neither beautiful nor fast, but I did finish. I knew I had completed something that would make me a better Nordic skier, and as I exited the course and caught my breath, I not so gracefully threw up my breakfast.

LET GO OF PERFECTION,
EVEN IF BREAKFAST BECOMES A PROJECTION.

Name That Loser

Think life is easy? Think all the folks who have been successful have just skipped their ways to the pots of gold? To put things in perspective, let's play a game called *Name That Loser*. I will describe true, painful stories about failure and loss. You get to decide which story is about which protagonist. Are you ready?

This business leader failed out of college and then went on to co-own a failed business.

    a. Fred Smith

    b. Steve Jobs

    c. Bill Gates

As a young boy, this intellectual powerhouse was told that he was "too stupid to learn anything."

    a. Albert Einstein

    b. Charles Darwin

    c. Thomas Edison

After this musical act's first performance, the paraphrased feedback was: "You are not going anywhere."

    a. The Beatles

    b. Beethoven

    c. Elvis Presley

This public speaker had a panic attack in front of five million fans.

    a. Jesus

    b. Dan Quayle

    c. Dan Harris

This award-winning Hollywood icon was told early in his career, "Why don't you stop wasting people's time and go out and become a dishwasher or something?"

    a. Walt Disney

    b. Steven Spielberg

    c. Sidney Poitier

This entertainment icon was told early on that she/he "was not right for [the screen]."

    a. Fred Astaire

    b. Christopher Reeve

    c. Oprah Winfrey

He's a politician who flunked out of school not once, but twice.

    a. James Carville

    b. Abraham Lincoln

    c. Dick Cheney

This author was told that he/she was writing in genres that "do not sell."

    a. Jack Canfield

    b. J.K. Rowling

    c. Steven King

The correct answer in each case is C, but all these folks—As, Bs, and Cs—saw major failures and major success. Let's learn a little more about their experiences.

According to business lore, Fred Smith wrote a paper about his overnight package-delivery concept (the world's first such model) in business school and received a mere C from a doubtful professor. Steve Jobs dropped out of Oregon's Reed College after only one semester. He also quit one of his first jobs to backpack around India.

In terms of intellectual powerhouses, Albert Einstein didn't speak fluently until he was nine, causing teachers to think he was slow. He was also expelled from school for his rebellious nature. Charles Darwin certainly seemed to have *daddy issues*, as it is believed that his father told him he would amount to nothing more than a disgrace to his family and to himself.

In music, the Beatles were told after their first audition in 1962, "We don't like [your] sound, and guitar music is on the way out." Back in the 18th century, Beethoven was allegedly told by his music instructor that he was a hopeless composer.

The stakes are high in public speaking, but the threat of being thrown off a cliff is something few speakers experience. That is exactly what happened to Jesus when he went to speak in his hometown of Nazareth. Luke 4:28-29 describes a scene that would probably scare away most other public speakers for good: "All the people in the synagogue were furious when they heard this. They got up, drove him out of town, and took him to the brow of the hill on which the town was built, in order to throw him down the cliff."

The world cringed in 1992 when Vice President Dan Quayle, leading a spelling bee for sixth-grade students at a New Jersey elementary school, corrected 12-year-old William Figueroa; the child spelled *potato* on the blackboard, and Quayle made the boy add an unnecessary "e" at the word's end.

I was speechless when I learned that Walt Disney was fired from a Missouri newspaper for "not being creative enough." And my jaw dropped when I learned that Steven Spielberg, the director of some of my favorite movies, was rejected from his top-choice college three times due to poor grades in high school.

Hollywood is tough. The story goes that Fred Astaire was told after his first screen test, "Can't act. Can't sing. Balding. Can dance a little." There are no words to explain the obstacles Christopher Reeve had to overcome in his lifetime. After winning hearts in *Superman*, the avid equestrian was thrown from his horse in 1995 and became a quadriplegic. Despite the accident, before his death in 2004, he remained active and started the Christopher & Dana Reeve Foundation, which supports research to develop cures and treatments for paralysis patients.

James Carville's personal mission statement is supposedly along the lines of, "No one will ever accuse [me] of taking [myself] seriously." Carville was the chief campaign strategist for Bill Clinton's 1992 presidential campaign. You are probably familiar with the story of Abraham Lincoln; even so, it deserves mention in the arena of political failure and triumph. Born into poverty, Lincoln was faced with defeat throughout his life. He lost eight elections, twice failed in business, and suffered a nervous breakdown. We have the opportunity to recall not only his failures but his successes, every single time we look at a penny.

Jack Canfield, co-creator of the *Chicken Soup for the Soul* series, which has sold more than 500 million copies worldwide, was rejected by 144 publishers. I wonder if any of those naysayers wound up weeping into their soup bowls as they thought about the missed opportunity. J. K. Rowling, author of the *Harry Potter* series, was rejected by more than a dozen publishers and likely felt hopeless as she scraped by on waitress tips and public assistance. Maybe she was imagining her future success when she wrote Albus Dumbledore's line: "Happiness can be found, even in the darkest of times, if one only remembers to turn on the light."

EMBRACE IMPERFECTION.
FAILURES ARE MOMENTS FOR REFLECTION.

Stick to Your Core

Moments of failure are often the best reminders to return to your center or core. An animated speaker at a recent Sun Valley Wellness Festival urged us to find our strength from our core as she enacted a scene we all can relate to in our everyday lives: vacuuming our floors. Imagine you're in the kitchen, and you're pretty sure the cord can also reach to the living room, so you push a little further. You make it and then think, "Let's just get to the dining room while I'm at it." You're pulling the power cord further and further and then—*rrrrrrr*—the cord comes unplugged, and the vacuum stops.

That is exactly what happens to you when you stray too far from your core: You are figuratively unplugged from your power source. You must find a way to plug back in, and that means getting back to your center.

At Nurture, I have experienced that feeling of pushing beyond our core—often through adding programs, expanding too quickly, and getting into what's known as *mission creep* in the non-profit world—until the power goes down. Program quality diminishes. Satisfaction is lowered. It's time to return to our center.

We created Nurture as a grassroots organization to enable hands-on work by volunteers to improve the nutrition and health of families. At our core is a desire to work directly with participants and see the impact of our programs firsthand. We want to change the world from the inside out. We are mostly moms with unique skills and expertise who help each other while helping ourselves, making key changes to our own eating habits and experimenting with ways to cook healthy meals for our families. Our positive changes radiate outward to the schools we are connected to, the food pantries and social service agencies in our local neighborhoods, and the people we believe we can help in a hands-on way. Our programs have been hugely successful because we are all so passionate about the work we are doing. We love the creative process and watching the participants in the programs come back each week with more stories about how they are changing their lives for the better.

But it wasn't always this way. In its first decade, Nurture grew exponentially and experienced growing pains consistent with such rapid expansion. Our leaders were spending less time with participants and more in meetings, preparing complex procedural documentation, and following bureaucratic processes. We were losing invaluable board members in droves because we had stopped having fun. The quality of our programs dipped. The farther we strayed from our core, the weaker we became.

All the while, my weekly ski lessons were teaching me about the importance of a strong core. Every top athlete will tell you that all power comes from a strong center. How many times did I need to hear that fact until I realized it was the answer for my struggles in my professional life?

Regardless of how many people had to say it and in how many ways, I finally got the message loud and clear and started the process of getting Nurture back to its core. We centralized our complex organization. We simplified our mission statement, focused on key programs, and found the fun again. I am proud to say that Nurture has recently received some of the best program feedback we have had in years, and I'm particularly proud of all the wonderful people who have had a hand in producing our success.

NO SUCH THING AS PERFECTION.
FAILURES POINT US IN THE RIGHT DIRECTION.

I'm Not Perfect, and Neither Are You

As a nutrition educator, I have failed in just about every setting. In class with participants, I have taught lessons that have gone over like a lead balloon. At home, I have made plenty of mistakes with my family, from cooking disasters to parenting *faux pas*. I have had moments when I've felt out of balance and have not been the poster child of wellness. One of the titles I considered for this book was *I'm Not Perfect, and Neither Are You*. I continue to love the moment when I gave up on the concept of perfection and embraced the bumpy road to progress. I noticed that life started to get a whole lot more fun.

Games are powerful tools that can help us to let go of perfection and have a little fun. When I've failed with wellness and nutrition progress, games have helped me, my family, and the broader community in our efforts to:

- Try new healthy foods.
- Avoid addictive and dangerous food additives.
- Create healthy lunches.

**FAILURE CAN LEAD TO GAME CREATION.
JOIN ME IN THE "IMPERFECT" NATION.**

Try New Healthy Foods

"AAAAAAAH!" Alexander yelled as he ran from his room in a panic. We were moving some furniture around for spring cleaning, and he had walked in while we were just about to move his bookshelf.

"That's weird," I said to Jeff.

"He usually only does that scream-and-run thing when he is watching *Curious George*."

You know those moments in Curious George when the inevitable trouble is about to occur? That irresistible string dangling from the counter that you just know he will pull—to create a cascade of breakable items that will inevitably crash to the floor? The fate of all the pies left on the table when Curious George is left unattended in the dining room before the big party? The lion cage you just know he will open?

When these kinds of moments happened in the show, Alexander used to literally do a backflip over the couch and run from the TV room. He would then go screaming down the hall with his hands clamped over his ears because he was so afraid of the trouble that curious little monkey was going to get into. This happened at least several times an episode, yet Alexander still loved watching that show.

When we were rearranging Alexander's room, there was no Curious George in sight. Jeff and I gave each other a perplexed look as we got back to our spring cleaning. Alexander had a horizontal bookshelf that acted as a cubby holder for some stuffed animals he had outgrown. We needed to move it someplace else, so we lifted it together and moved it across the room.

Then we saw the stash. And we knew why the little monkey was running down the hall.

Under Alexander's bookshelf were about 600 kid-sized, omega-3 fish-oil pills. I had wanted the kids to try a regimen of these chewable pills, and I had told them simply that they had to eat them, two a day at breakfast. There was a year's worth of omega-3 pills that Alexander had hidden and told me he had eaten. We heard his bare feet pattering down the stairs as he continued to flee the scene of the crime.

"I guess we need to find another way to get omega-3s into Alexander," Jeff said to me as he went to find a garbage bag.

LEARN FROM YOUR MISTAKES, EVEN AS THE CURIOUS MONKEY ESCAPES.

Bingo!

Do you know that it can take as many as 16 exposures to a food for our taste buds to get used to a flavor? That means that you should not give up too early when encouraging an expanded palate for you or your kids. However, forcing food tastings is a recipe for failure. What I started to do after the bookshelf incident was to create a weekly bingo card, with food instead of numbers in the squares. I would write the names of foods that my kids had not yet tried, like parsley, Brussels sprouts, or Swiss chard. One week, I filled it simply with all of the varieties of lettuce we were growing in our garden. Over time, Alexander chose lots of omega-3-rich foods, like salmon, tuna, walnuts, and flax seeds, from his bingo card, instead of taking the pills. Once the cards were set up, I told my kids that they should put an X on the squares that named a food they had tried that week. A *bingo* was complete when they made a line of X's diagonally, horizontally, or vertically. Since they didn't have to fill in the entire card, the game gave them choices, and it made trying new foods fun. I even came up with small prizes, including special excursions or events that the children had wanted. (Note: Prizes should *not* be candy.)

Elena and Alexander's interest in trying new foods skyrocketed. And you'll never guess what Alexander's favorite food is today: salmon, rich in omega-3. He also learned about his favorite grain, quinoa, through this game.

Test out versions of bingo in your own home. Keep trying and don't give up. Maybe you will need to think of incentives for trying new foods yourself. If you are searching for more resources, the Iowa Department of Public Health maintains a website called Pick a Better Snack*. You can access its pre-made monthly bingo cards, which also encourage physical activity.

HAVE FUN AND TRY NEW BITES.
AVOID FOOD-RELATED FIGHTS.

Avoid Addictive and Dangerous Food Additives

Alexander isn't our only kid to have gotten busted during spring cleaning. One year, at the bottom of Elena's dresser drawer, we found a huge stash of all of the candies we had told our kids to avoid: Starbursts, jelly beans, Gobstoppers, gummy bears, and sticky lollipops. I had been preaching to the kids about the dangers of food coloring, but I had been using terms they not only didn't know but also couldn't care less about.

- "Some food additives are actually neurotoxins!"
- "The yellow food dye Tartrazine has been banned in European countries, but our country still uses it!"
- "I read today that food dyes might be linked to the increase in Attention Deficit Disorder!"

Jeff and I looked down at the cesspool of food coloring in Elena's drawer. At that moment, she walked into the room.

"That's *mine*!" she screamed, pointing to the drawer.

*For information about this program, including monthly bingo cards, see www.idph.state.ia.us/inn/PickABetterSnack.aspx

These chemical-laden candies had become valuable com-
modities to our daughter. I knew that being the *candy police*
would make matters even worse, so I tried out *candy lawyer*
and started negotiations.

"I know you've been saving up for that new Polly Pocket set,"
I said in as calm a voice as I could muster. (Polly Pocket toys are
small, plastic figures that come with accessories.)

"Yes," Elena said suspiciously.

"I'll buy this candy from you. A nickel for a small one and a
dime for a big one. I bet you have almost enough to buy that
Polly Pocket set you really want."

"A *quarter* for the big ones," Elena countered, and we made
a deal.

LEARN TO PUSH RESET.
BARTER FOR A POLLY POCKET SET.

Scavenger Hunt!

I would be absolutely broke if I continued to have to bribe
my kids for food-related compliance, so I was thrilled to learn
about an activity through Nurture called the Food Ingredient
Scavenger Hunt. There are infinite variations on this theme,
but the general idea is that you provide kids with a list of
things they need to find, and they get points for finding them.
When my kids were old enough to read, we started doing
scavenger hunts as an activity to teach them how to read food
labels. The genius of this game is that you are mixing in important lessons. As the participants find ingredients, you, of

course, provide them with some educational background about those ingredients.

My favorite example came after a discussion of how our pink yogurt, drinks, and ice cream get their color. None of us will forget that day.

"Time to leave!" Jeff said as he finished packing up the car. We were planning a trip to the Grand Canyon, and we had many hours of driving ahead of us, including stops for snacks at gas stations. I knew that gas stations were the best place to find all kinds of nasty food additives.

I started the game. "Okay, kids! Our first game is Food Ingredient Scavenger Hunt. You'll see the list of items on the first sheet in the activity packet I just handed you."

"There are *bugs* in our food?" Elena asked. She is a fast reader.

"Yes! You are going to be looking for the word 'carmine' at our first gas stop. First one to find it gets five points!"

"Gross, Mom! The sheet says that carmine is made of cochineal extract from the female *Dactylopius coccus costa.*" Her voice began to rise. "They are harvested mainly in Peru and the Canary Islands. The girl bugs eat pink cactus pads, and the color gathers in their bodies and eggs. Once harvested, dried, and ground, these bugs make their way into things like yogurt, frozen fruit bars, fruit filling, and fruit juice."

Alexander wanted to one-up his sister. "So what? A little bug juice never hurt anyone."

"Alexander! It says that carmine can cause allergic reactions in some people." We got to our first gas station shop. To the dismay of all the customers, and certainly the guy working behind the counter, my kids ran in the door yelling, "Dead bugs! We're on the lookout for dead bugs!"

Elena was the winner of this round. She emerged from the gas station with a plastic wrapped cookie—Grandma's brand—in her hands. She was very proud of her find. She held on to that cookie for dear life throughout the entire round trip as it crumbled inside of the packaging. She was excited to show the bug cookie to her friends and teacher when she returned home.

"I can't believe Grandma put dead bugs in her cookies," Jeff said as we drove past that same gas station on the way back from the Grand Canyon.

"Yeah, Mom. We'll stick with your homemade ones for now on," my kids said to me as I smiled stealthily in the front seat.

**HAVE A GAME OF TRY-AND-FIND-ITS.
BEWARE OF GAS STATION RIOTS.**

Create Healthy Lunches

One of the most difficult transitions our family had when changing from a Montessori school to the local public schools in the Chicago suburbs was what to eat for lunch. At Montessori, all the parents sent packed lunches, and no sweets were allowed. When we signed up for public schools, I was pleased to hear that the school had a cafeteria where my kids could get lunch every day. No more packing lunches in the morning! But my smile faded when I got my first statement from the school district:

1/15/09   a la carte brownie ($2), a la carte cookie ($1.50)   total $3.50

1/16/09   a la carte brownie ($2), a la carte cookie ($1.50)   total $3.50

1/17/09   a la carte brownie ($2), a la carte cookie ($1.50)   total $3.50

1/18/09   a la carte brownie ($2), a la carte cookie ($1.50)   total $3.50

1/19/09   a la carte brownie ($2), a la carte cookie ($1.50)   total $3.50

1/22/09   a la carte brownie ($2), a la carte cookie ($1.50)   total $3.50

1/23/09   a la carte brownie ($2), a la carte cookie ($1.50)   total $3.50

1/24/09   a la carte brownie ($2), a la carte cookie ($1.50)   total $3.50

1/25/09   a la carte brownie ($2), a la carte cookie ($1.50)   total $3.50

1/26/09   a la carte brownie ($2), a la carte cookie ($1.50)   total $3.50

I tried not to be upset with Alexander as I asked him what he usually did at lunchtime.

"Well, we go through this line and take what we want. Then, there is a checkout lady at the end."

"Did she ever say anything to you about how you were just getting a cookie and a brownie?"

"Um, no," Alexander said.

Whether this was the truth or not, I will never know. But, thanks to watching Nurture's educator Juliette work with kids, I was seasoned to know that punishment and forced action were not the way to go. I needed to figure out a way to empower Alexander to make good decisions on his own.

LEARN TO EMPOWER WITH CHOICE.
THE LUNCH LADY MAY NOT USE HER VOICE.

Grade That Lunch!

I contacted Alexander's teacher the next morning and asked if I could do a free nutrition lesson in his grade the following week.

"Sure!" she said. "I have been wanting to do something about the quality of my kids' lunches. In the afternoon, I can tell the difference between who's had a good lunch and who hasn't."

So I showed up with the game: Grade That Lunch.

"I'm going to show you a series of lunch boxes, and you will give each lunch a score. Each food group included gets a point. The highest score possible is a five. You get one point for having each of the following: whole grain, protein, dairy/calcium, fruits, and veggies. Are you ready?"

"*Yes!*"

So I put up the first picture of a lunch.

Lunch menu example #1:
- French fries and ketchup
- Power drink or soda
- Candy bar

There was a pause as the kids tried to reconcile the food groups with the picture. A little girl raised her hand. "Is it possible to get a zero?"

"Yes! That's right. This lunch is a *zero*."

Then we moved on to the next picture.

Lunch menu example #2:
- Hamburger on white bun
- Tater tots and ketchup

- Chocolate chip cookie
- Sweetened iced tea

The kids studied the photo.

"One?"

"You got it. We can count the hamburger meat as protein. Harvard's Healthy Eating Plate mentions that white potatoes don't count as a veggie, and the fried aspect of the tater tots renders them unhealthy. Let's move on to another lunch!"

Lunch menu example #3:

- Enriched crackers
- Cheese and ham
- Reese's Peanut Butter Cup
- Sour candies

"I think a two," a voice came from the back of the room.

"Yes, we are moving up."

The meat on the picture was not particularly appetizing, but we decided to count it as protein. The cheese earned a point for dairy.

"What about a point for the crackers as whole grains?" another voice questioned.

"Nope. The word 'enriched' gives away the fact that the grains have been processed and are no longer whole. Let's move on."

Lunch menu example #4:

- Tuna salad on enriched bread
- Cherry tomatoes and cucumbers

- Clementine
- Pretzels
- Pickles
- Cake

"Hmmm," I heard.

"I think we are moving up to a three. I see a fruit, veggies, and protein," said a child in the first row.

"How could you make this lunch even better?"

We brainstormed and decided that exchanging the enriched bread with whole grain bread would be good. We could also omit the pretzels or forgo the cake and have the clementine for dessert.

I noticed Alexander taking in all of the discussion among his classmates, despite not saying anything himself. He was hearing from his friends what a *cool* lunch was.

Lunch menu example #5:
- Chicken salad in whole-wheat pita
- Red pepper, carrots, hummus
- Greek yogurt and fresh berries
- Whole-grain/veggie pasta salad

"FIVE! FIVE!" The kids were all now really excited and were shouting.

"I see chicken for protein!"

"Hummus, too!"

"Whole grains in the pita!"

"Calcium in the Greek yogurt!"

"Fruits *and* veggies!"

The teacher helped me to calm the class. Then, we talked about how delicious the *five* lunch looked.

A few weeks later, Alexander's teacher called me with good news and bad news.

"The good news is that the kids' lunches are improving a ton. I'm seeing a noticeable change in attention and attitude after lunch. Thank you, Kathryn."

"You're welcome. What's the bad news?"

"Well, the principal had to intervene in the lunch room a few times these last two weeks. He had heard tons of noise and wanted to know why there were numbers being screamed from the lunchroom and echoing down the halls."

"What was going on?"

"I think the kids just got a little overexcited about being able to assign their *own grades* at school."

LET THE KIDS YELL AND SHOUT.
A GREAT LUNCH IS WHAT THEY'RE EXCITED ABOUT.

Be Playful as You Push the Reset Button

To be able to absorb the lessons our failures can teach us, it is important to incorporate an appropriate mood of playfulness into our work, whether our activities take place at home, at the office, or anywhere else. Playfulness allows us to override the reptilian part of our brains (that controls our reactionary fight-or-flight responses) and get our prefrontal cortex, the logic center, back online.

In my early days of consulting, I took myself so incredibly seriously because I felt that I needed to prove my value. With all those unnecessary fight-or-flight biochemicals (cortisol and adrenaline) in my system, I was a ball of tension waiting to explode. What I learned later in life, through my ski lessons, is that a bit of play can do amazing things to push the *reset button* and transform fear into success. Playfulness can often do wonders when creating an environment of productivity and efficiency. Top executives and athletes manage stress and reset with techniques that are as simple as taking a break to go for a walk, sharing a funny joke, or listening to an inspirational piece of music that will prompt a smile or the relaxation response.

The U.S. Nordic Ski Team used a particularly effective method to push the reset button right before the high-pressure 2015 World Championships. Under great stress, everyone was preparing for the big competition. When the coach challenged his skiers to make a music video incorporating choreographed moves and a fun, modern song, their initial response was, "We don't have time for this!" But with the persistence and insistence of the coach, the team selected the song "Uptown Funk" and started to put together some cool dance moves. A subtle shift in the team's mood came at first, but before long, all were embracing their inner (non-professional) performers and striking fun and powerful poses*.

While Nordic skiing is a technical sport in which small movements make a big difference, the team let loose with the dance

* To watch the video, which has been viewed by over one million viewers, you can go to: www.healthysolutionsofsv. com/push-reset-button/

moves and was able to disconnect from the idea that perfection was the goal. What they learned is that often when you take away the need to be perfect, playfulness will move in and make itself at home. The team's spirit skyrocketed to an all-time high. The citizens of Falun, Sweden, where the championships were held, were thrilled to see scenes from their hometown in the video. As the U.S. athletes walked down the streets of Falun, they were met with cheers wherever they went. As one Swede said, "Americans are such awesome people; they always come up with something creative and fun!"

It's pretty impressive that they came home with some medals, too.

GET FUNKY AND SING OUT LOUD.
MAKE YOUR ENTIRE NATION PROUD.

A Falling Win in Poland

Over and over, as I talk to Olympians, I hear stories of incredible recovery while facing certain defeat. One story that stands out vividly is from Kikkan Randall, four-time Olympic Nordic skier and current member of the U.S. Ski Team.

"We were in Poland, doing sprint races, which means that I had already put in a lot of effort just to qualify for the race I was in. I was in the next heat and ready to go through my next trial. The gun goes off, and I'm putting everything I've got into the current round. But then … another skier skied right over the tops of my skis and we were both down, a jumble of skis and poles and legs and spandexed bodies. Since the sprint was only a few minutes, I could have said to myself at that moment that I was done; the race was over. But for some reason, I decided to get up and finish the race, just for me."

Kikkan got up and rejoined the race, powered by adrenaline and love of the sport. She not only caught the pack, but passed it.

She continues, "Just as I was about 20 meters from the end, I realized that my legs had turned to Jell-O and could only do so much to keep this superhuman pace going. Two other skiers passed me just at the finish by a ski-length, but I was amazed to have finished third. I was thrilled that I had done this race for myself, but I had pulled through ultimately for my team."

At dinner that night, a huge swarm of people arrived, and murmurs and excitement rippled through the crowd. The skiers heard something about the Polish president having arrived to give special recognition to a skier with whom he was particularly impressed.

Kikkan recalls, "All of a sudden, I was asked to stand to receive a great honor and symbol of Poland, a huge 45-pound purple geode [rock] that represented the courage and strength that I had demonstrated by getting up and finishing strong in a race that I could have potentially never started. I stood and beamed in the spotlight with the Polish president."

Later, Kikkan would learn that the presenter of the award was the president of a Polish *radio station*, not the president of Poland, an important distinction. But that didn't diminish the pride that she felt in placing third in this race because she was able to transform defeat into success through her love of the sport.

IF YOU FALL, JUST LET GO.
GET AN AWARD FROM THE KING OF POLISH RADIO.

Bullfighters and Teflon

"What is the worst thing that can happen? Is the client going to kill you!?"

Our young team of consultants, sleep deprived and pumped up on caffeine after a hard push to prepare the final presentation for our client, was having a collective panic attack before a big presentation. I am sure that this dynamic had something to do with the fact that perfectionism had leaked into the project work plan. We had worked into all hours of the night, tweaking every last bullet point, until I finally lost my patience, and declared as I walked out the door, "Perfection is the opposite of ... *GET IT DONE!*"

So it got done, but everyone was nervous as we re-grouped the next day right before the big meeting. It was a bit of a fret-fest, until our managing partner, Bob, showed up. Bob was always relaxed and unruffled, despite stories of some pretty tough client meetings. So we nicknamed him Teflon Bob because everything seemed to slide right off.

"Guys, you are consultants, not matadors. These are clients, not bulls. Relax and put things into perspective."

He was right. Our team was spending so much time in fight-or-flight mode that our central nervous systems were on overload. This level of stress was completely inappropriate for the reality we faced. Like Bob said, we were not in mortal danger. We were, however, hurting our chances of delivering a high-quality presentation. When the fight-or-flight response kicks in, your prefrontal cortex, the brain center responsible for executive function, goes offline—not the best circumstances under which to make a compelling, rational, and logical argument.

I had seen a real matador in action while studying in Mexico during an exchange program. It was a small-town bullfight, and there was an amateur sense about the whole thing, except that the bull was real, enormous, and furious. The local setting perhaps explained why there were no protections in place for the matador. This amateur bullfight also lacked the artistry and gracefulness that you might see at a professional bullfight. There was, instead, a lot of running around and panic, and the bull eventually succeeded in goring the matador, jabbing his horn right through the poor guy's thigh. As the bull galloped around furiously with the matador flopping on him like a rag doll, the flight response spread to the crowd, and everyone evacuated the first few rows of the stands.

I was horrified, but my local companions seemed to think it was all fine and well.

"Come on, we don't want to miss the post-fight reception!" said one.

This meet-and-greet session with the gored matador actually took place. The matador, a gaping hole in his leg, stood and took pictures with all the fans who came up to shake his hand. I have my picture with him hanging on my wall. The photo* serves to

* If you are interested in seeing this photo, please visit this site (I've also put a picture of a non-life threatening scene from my days in management consulting): www.healthysolution-sofsv.com/fight-flight/

remind me that I must distinguish when I'm truly in danger from when I should let the situation and associated stress slide right off, just as Teflon Bob advised.

MAKE THE MOST OF YOUR FAN RECEPTION, EVEN IF YOU RISK A LEG INFECTION.

Mantra #5: Embrace the yard sale is a reminder to make the most of failures in your life. Try not to take yourself so seriously and learn how to pick yourself up from mistakes in order to learn from them. Know that a little cod liver oil is actually good for you and will make you stronger. Remember to stick to your core because, when you act from a place of center, you have the most power. This concept of core power is true in skiing, life, and wellness. In all of the subjects of classroom Earth, it is important to be playful. Remember that the methods through which you successfully address failures can often be in the form of games. We saw hidden omega-3 fish pills lead to bingo, drawers full of candy turn into a scavenger hunt, and a lunch disaster turn into Grade That Lunch. Just because you're a grown up doesn't mean you can't act like a kid again. When you experience failure in your life, remember to be willing to press the reset button and continue ahead with a good attitude. *Embrace the yard sale* is about falling down, getting up, and learning from and laughing through the process.

ACTION ITEMS FROM THIS CHAPTER

FOR SUCCESS IN LIFE:

- Learn from your mistakes. Remember that the most successful people in life have had some of the biggest failures.
- Stick to your core. Recognize that failures can be an important signal that you may have strayed too far from your center.
- Be playful. Don't take yourself too seriously.

FOR SUCCESS ON THE SLOPES:

- Take some cod liver oil from time to time. That might mean doing some training that pushes you harder than you'd like.
- Remember the fun in the sport. Enjoy your losses as much as your wins.
- Rest and play are underrated. Yes, even before a big competition, you have time for both.

FOR SUCCESS IN WELLNESS:

- Understand failure as the process of leading you toward better wellness.
- Give up the concept of being perfect and instead embrace yourself as a beautiful work of art, always in the process of heading toward balance.
- Learn from your failures and even create positive games from such experiences. Examples include bingo, scavenger hunts, and Grade That Lunch.

Mantra #6
Throw Yourself Down the Mountain

Do or do not. There is no try.

—YODA

from Star Wars: The Empire Strikes Back

What I love about skiing is that it forces you to let go and let gravity help you. As you move into a turn, it is essential that you release your weight down the mountain, letting the edges of the skis flatten so that you can cruise smoothly. Before living in the mountains, I would hear the phrase "just let go" and wonder, *how*? With skiing, you practice the art of letting go every single time you turn. It reminds me of what Baron Baptiste wrote in *Journey Into Power* about *trying hard*, which "invites strain and struggle," and *trying easy*, which "gives you the levity and freedom to fly." This yoga-ism holds true when skiing. Trying easy means learning to make a commitment to the natural forces of nature. Being afraid creates struggle, and struggle creates more fear. Getting past fear opens up the possibility of skiing with ease and grace, almost like dancing. The feeling I get when I am skiing with freedom is a sensation that is the closest to what I imagine it feels like to fly—exhilarating.

From Bunny Hills to Double Black Diamonds

Swish, swish went the snow as we swooped down the bowls. On these ungroomed black diamond runs, only the most confident and skilled skiers can be found. Jeff had stopped ahead and was looking back up the slope at me, his mouth gaping in happy surprise as I swooped down to meet him with great confidence and a big smile.

"I'm channeling my inner Jedi!" I answered his unspoken question.

"You are a great, confident skier. What have you done with my wife?"

It was the end of my fourth season living in Sun Valley and skiing on Baldy. I had learned to approach something scary with a positive attitude. I had set my foundation in my feet and put in many, many hours in my ski boots—both alpine and Nordic—over the past four years. I had set my vision to understand the *why* driving all of this hard work and what it would feel like when I finally got there. I had taken my vision and broken it down into small but manageable goals that I measured and tracked. I had failed and fallen many times and would certainly again, but I knew to learn from these experiences so that I would continue to improve.

I was now focused on the final ingredient: complete engagement. It also happened to be the focus of one of my lessons with extreme skier Danielle, the co-head coach of the DIVAS program.

"Kathryn, you have to throw yourself down the mountain!" Danielle said to me, as she smiled and critiqued my last few turns. "Gravity is your friend when you're on skis. You have to commit as you make your turn. You've got the technique. You've got the upper and lower body separation. If you position your body down the mountain, your skis will come with you. You have to trust."

I was about to whine about how scary the terrain looked—Danielle liked to find the hardest and most unexplored terrain in the bowls—but I stopped. I looked out over the beautiful landscape and thought about what my kids had said on last Sunday's movie night. We had watched *Star Wars: The Empire Strikes Back* for the hundredth time. "Mom, Luke thinks Yoda is crazy," said Alexander.

"Luke is a whiner," added Elena. "Look at how he rolls his eyes when Yoda asks him to do something hard." Luke was unsuccessfully trying to channel the force to lift his X-wing fighter out of the murky pond on Dagobah using only his mind. "You get mad at me if I roll *my* eyes!" Elena said defensively, looking at me.

She was right. Luke was not focusing on the present moment, and he believed that the exercise Yoda was asking him to do was impossible; therefore, it was. He needed to commit to completing his task fully instead of second-guessing himself or thinking his 800-year-old mentor was senile.

I snapped back to the present moment in the bowls of Baldy. I smiled at my lucid and much more youthful than Yoda mentor, Danielle, and swooped down the bowls, committing at every turn.

ENGAGE 100 PERCENT.
COMMIT FULLY ON YOUR DESCENT.

Commit to Facing Fear

Throwing yourself down the mountain means staying forward on your skis. Staying forward can often mean getting out of your comfort zone. When we get in situations that we feel are extremely challenging, our natural reflex is to recoil and protect. On skis, that protective reflex means getting your weight *into the backseat* (i.e., your butt), which can set you up for a crash. Why? Because when your weight is on the tails of your skis, you are simply propelled faster as you speed further out of balance. You eventually will fall or run into something if you sit in the backseat.

In business and life, getting out of your comfort zone is critical to success. One of the things that people fear most is public speaking, and I have had to do my share of it in my role as the executive director at Nurture. Speaking to inform and entertain is one thing, but giving a talk to ask for large sums of money to ensure the sustainability of the organization is another. Stakes are high. The pressure is intense. Few people like being asked for money; and even fewer enjoy asking. I was thinking about an upcoming presentation that I had for a large grant, and I decided to ask my kids what they thought.

"Be prepared," the always-organized and mature Elena said.

Good point. That kid has got her head on straight, I thought. *But I was prepared! What am I so afraid of? I just didn't feel ready.*

"You really love what you do, don't you, Mom?" asked Alexander.

A profound yes would be the answer to that question. At Nurture, I help kids and parents live healthier and happier lives through our education programs. I teach and direct classes, follow up on program results, and work on strategy—all things I love to do. The job is flexible and allows me to be the best version of myself. I always love hearing how we've changed peoples' lives for the better.

"Focus on the love," Alexander continued. "The last time I was really, really scared was right before the pond skim at Dollar Dayz. Love got me through."

The pond skim is the end-of-the-ski-season celebration at Dollar Mountain, the same mountain where I had learned to ski with those little booger-laden four-year-olds. Since that time, the Sun Valley Company completely transformed the place, building a beautiful lodge and adding all kinds of cool features to the ski mountain, including terrain parks, major jumps, and an Olympic-sized half pipe. The entire town gathers there on the last day of the season to celebrate our amazing ski town. The highlight of the event is a pond skim, where people tuck their bodies low on their skis and speed down the lower half of the mountain, trying to make it across a pond of icy water at the bottom of the hill. Participants in costume get a discounted entry fee, so everyone is decked out in fun and outrageous outfits, all certain to get soaked. The event involves great bravery, especially considering the highly visible line of ambulances and ski patrol, ready with stretchers and snorkels.

"I was at the very start of the run, and I felt the butterflies go crazy in my stomach. I almost wanted to turn back," Alexander recounted.

As his mother, I was also extremely nervous before he started his descent. I remember looking for him from the bottom of the hill, with butterflies raging in my own stomach. As I spotted him in his bright superman cape, I thought to myself, "Is he really going to do this?"

Alexander continued his recollection: "Right before I almost backed out, I thought to myself, 'Wait! I *love* skiing. And I love going super fast and doing tricks. This is my *thing!*'"

So Alexander took off from the top of the hill with a huge smile on his face. He sped down the mountain and across and into the pond. He didn't make it all the way across that first year, but he emerged soaking wet, grinning, and proud of himself, full of love for the sport.

He has gone back year after year, perfecting his technique. This past year, his costume (a sort of creepy-looking Blue Man Group suit) stayed dry as he whisked across like a pro.

Now, whenever I have to give a presentation that might scare me, I think about Alexander on his first run on Dollar Dayz.

COMMIT AND BE BOLD.
DUNK IN A POND THAT'S FREEZING COLD.

Transform Fear into Love

The idea of connecting with love when you are afraid seemed intuitive to my son, but it is not yet a widely used tool in the business world or for most people in their daily endeavors. Dr. David Hawkins contends in his groundbreaking book *Power vs. Force* that more than 85 percent of humans calibrate below a positive level on his map of consciousness. Let me define my understanding of what Hawkins' map of consciousness is. I will warn you that I'm going into woo-woo territory (again), but I really like how his work sends the message that we need to move out of shame, apathy, and fear and into courage, joy, and love to experience the best in life.

Hawkins used calibration of neuromuscular testing (often called applied kinesiology) on thousands of people until he came up with a scale that mapped the spectrum of emotions, from those that make us the weakest to those that make us the strongest. His map of consciousness ranges from a low of 20 (shame) to a high of 1,000 (enlightenment). To give you a sense of the ends of the spectrum, 20 is near self-destruction and 700 to 1,000 is where folks like Jesus, Krishna, and Buddha register.

Now, let's take a look at the difference between love and fear.

> 20 – Shame
> 30 – Guilt
> 50 – Apathy
> 75 – Grief
> **100 – Fear**
> 125 – Desire
> 150 – Anger
> 175 – Pride
> 200 – Courage
> > this is the turning point at which emotions make you stronger versus weaker
> 250 – Neutrality
> 310 – Willingness
> 350 – Acceptance
> 400 – Reason
> **500 – Love**

540 – Joy

600 – Peace

700 to 1,000 – Enlightenment

Love is 400 points above fear on the map of consciousness, well beyond the tipping point at which emotions start to help instead of hurt you (at 200). When you are in a place of love, you are not only able to be stronger in your endeavors, you are also attracting other positive people, ideas, and beliefs. This higher emotion of love is in direct contrast to being in a state of fear, when you are weaker and attract negative people, ideas, and beliefs. No wonder Alexander has made it safely and triumphantly through several years of pond skims. He is starting from a place of love. And when I received that large grant that contributed greatly to the sustainability of Nurture, I knew that it was love that had made me strong.

TRANSFORM FEAR INTO LOVE.
FEEL YOUR STRENGTH RISE ABOVE.

Commit to Finding Purpose

Sun Valley is a community that vibrates at a high level on the map of consciousness, in my opinion. People simply seem to have a great deal of acceptance, love, joy, and peace in this community. Whether or not this has to do with a higher reading on the scale, what I can say with certainty is that this location has one of the highest densities of non-profit work that I have seen. In a small valley with a population of less than

20,000, there are several hundred thriving non-profit organizations that make peoples' lives better every day. We have a food pantry that provides access to some of the healthiest food I have encountered in hunger relief (The Hunger Coalition); organizations that work with individuals and veterans with disabilities to allow them to experience the joy of alpine skiing and outdoor adventures (Higher Ground); and a community YMCA that offers, among its many life-enhancing programs, free swim lessons to every child*.

Most importantly, this community embraces the concept that volunteerism is good for your health and well-being. Numerous studies show increased life spans for those who participate in altruistic activities. I have seen the results play out across town. When I finish the Sun Valley Half Marathon or compete in a Nordic race, I notice that many of the folks that kick my butt are twice my age.

FIND YOUR PURPOSE ON PLANET EARTH.
KNOW HOW MUCH EACH OF US IS WORTH.

Don't Be a Squirrel

"Mommy! Look how cute it is!" said Elena, our family's animal lover. She was pointing at a grey squirrel that had run down a tree and was crossing the road. We were taking Elena to the park in a Baby Jogger stroller when she was just a toddler.

---

* For more information about how the Wood River Valley is cultivating a young generation of philanthropists, please visit Wow Students at www.wow-students.org/

"Daddy, he's crossing the street! And there is a car!" said Elena with concern. Oh, no. The squirrel did that thing where it makes a choice and runs one way, then changes its mind and runs in the opposite direction, then back again. As it continued to second-guess itself, the car got closer and closer and closer.

Splat!

We turned our eyes away in horror.

"WAAHHHHHHHHHH!!" screamed Elena.

We pushed the stroller away from the scene of the crime as fast as we could. I knew we had a terrible day in front of us. Elena was heartbroken to see harm come even to the tiniest of ants. We knew the squirrel episode could be scarring for life.

"Stupid squirrel," said Jeff under his breath.

"If only he could have just made up its mind!"

MAKE UP YOUR MIND AND BE BOLD.
DON'T GO SPLAT IN THE MIDDLE OF THE ROAD.

The Squirrel Effect

It can be embarrassing to be in the field of nutrition in this day and age. We are a nation of squirrels ourselves, changing our minds over and over again about what is the right way to go. Low calorie? Higher calorie? Low fat? High fat? Low carb? High carb? Meat eating? Vegetarian? The contrasting list goes on and on. Nutritionists have given so much conflicting advice that we have confused the population and put them at as much risk as a clan of confused squirrels trying to cross a multilane highway. I am afraid that if we don't commit and engage with a solution, we will all go *splat* as well!

Nutritional advice, in an official form—beyond what parents or grandparents teach about healthy eating—has been around for just over a century. The U.S. Department of Agriculture (USDA) published its first nutrition guidelines in 1894. These guidelines originated as a simple farmers' bulletin, but the advice continued to grow from there. What is most confusing to me about how that advice evolved over the 20th century is that, even as the problem being addressed changed so dramatically, our nation did not consider that we might need to change the source of our advice. In the first half of the century, which included the Great Depression and two World Wars, the problem was that we simply did not have enough food. One of the primary reasons soldiers were turned away from military service was because they were malnourished. The National School Lunch Program, also run by the USDA, began in 1946 as a way to reach children who might otherwise not have access to adequate nutrition. Having the Department of Agriculture involved at this point, when the focus was addressing inadequate nutrition, made perfect sense.

As the 20th century came to a close, however, the problem was no longer one of adequate calories. In 2005, the *New England Journal of Medicine* reported that, for the first time in American history, today's children may be the first to have a shorter average lifespan than their parents due to the health-related impact of obesity and nutritionally linked diseases. The problem has shifted so dramatically that more soldiers are now turned away from military service for being overweight than underweight. Health care costs have skyrocketed into the trillions of dollars to address nutritionally related diseases. The crazy thing is that food insecurity and malnutrition still exist! Thanks to the USDA, we have a flood of corn and starchy products in our food system, providing plenty of calories while lacking nutritional balance. Because starchy foods are plentiful and cheap, the lower-income population is disproportionally affected by obesity. Food distribution lines across the nation are full of the malnourished and overfed.

LOOKING ONLY TO THE USDA FOR ADVICE, OUR NATION COULD PAY A DEAR PRICE.

Time for a New Opinion

Let's say that your car doesn't seem to be working well. It is sputtering and clanking and doesn't seem safe to drive. You have always brought it to your favorite mechanic because he seems to understand how to fix whatever mechanical problem might be at play. He has his standard set of tools, and he loves to use them. You hesitate going back this time, however, because you have a sense that the problem has nothing to do with the car itself but instead with the gas that you are putting into it. You've always bought your gas from that same favorite mechanic because it's what he recommends. So, where do you go now?

The USDA is the old-school mechanic. The standard tools are its subsidy programs. Who is the broken down car in this metaphor? You! Your kids! Your friends and family! If you are interested in learning more about the USDA and its role in the food chain, I encourage you to watch *Fed Up*, the 2014 documentary by executive producers Katie Couric and Laurie David.

When I met Dr. David Katz, co-founder and director of Yale University's Prevention Research Center and founder of the Turn the Tide Foundation, he revealed a statistic that shocked me to the core. Up to 80 percent of deaths are triggered by lifestyle and eating choices. I knew that the number was high, but 80 percent? I am not a particularly morbid person, but I have looked up the leading causes of death in the U.S. at various points in the last decade. Heart disease and cancer, easily linked to nutrition, always stay at the top. Today, as I go through the rest of the list, I see that 8 out of 10 of the causes are strongly linked to nutrition. I am amazed that Alzheimer's disease, referred to by some preventive health practitioners as "Type 3 diabetes," has moved up to the sixth leading cause of death.

Based on the sad state of American wellness, it's clear that the federal government is not the best source of information and guidance. Enter the plethora of nutritional experts that rose to fill the void in the second half of the 20th century. Returning to our car metaphor, let's refer to this group as the *fuel evaluators*. Rather than taking the mechanic's point of view and trying to repair the car, they will evaluate the various options in terms of what you put in your tank. The problem we encounter with fuel evaluators is that they often have conflicting advice. How can you decide what to do?

In this chapter, I will provide a recap of my experiences on the spectrum of fuel evaluation experts. I will add that Katz is one of my favorite fuel evaluators of all time because he makes a point to keep his messaging as positive as possible. He involves his family in the process, working with his wife on the *Nutrition Detectives* curriculum and with his kids on *UnJunk Yourself*, a library of music videos that teaches adolescents about health. His mission in life is to turn the tide away from obesity and poor nutrition so that we can move towards optimal health and wellness.

TIME FOR A NEW GUIDE.
HELP OUR NATION TURN THE TIDE.

Diet Is a Four-Letter Word

I have personally tried many diets, from the Scarsdale Diet to the Atkins Diet to the South Beach Diet. While I appreciated some great advice from the doctors behind these diets, I was often left confused or unable to keep up the plan for very long. As I was studying for my certification in nutritional counseling, I was exposed to new theories and advice on nutrition that expanded my view on food and its role in wellness. I learned to drop the word *diet* and replace it with *lifestyle*. Some of my favorite books on a healthy eating lifestyle include:

- Dr. Andrew Weil's *Eating Well for Optimum Health: The Essential Guide to Bringing Health and Pleasure Back to Eating*
- Dr. Walter Willett's *Eat, Drink, and Be Healthy: The Harvard Medical School Guide to Healthy Eating*
- Paul Pitchford's *Healing with Whole Foods: Asian Traditions and Modern Nutrition*
- Jamie Oliver's *Jamie At Home: Cook Your Way to the Good Life*
- FairShare CSA Coalition's *From Asparagus to Zucchini: A Guide to Cooking Farm-Fresh Seasonal Produce*

- Tanya Wenman Steel and Tracey Seaman's *Real Food for Healthy Kids*

While these books and more helped me replace the concept of dieting with that of lifestyle change, diet advice continued to pile up from every corner of the globe. As is human nature, I was intrigued by the new trends: macrobiotic, the Zone, paleo, primal, vegan, raw, raw vegan, and so on. These concepts all seemed really cool! But how can I avoid becoming a squirrel, running in a frenzy from one fad to the next?

The key to overcoming the squirrel effect is to know that you have your own answer to your own winning eating plan right inside of you. It's called your gut, now beginning to be referred to as our *second brain*. What each of us needs to do is tap into the innate ability of the body to send us signals about when we are making good decisions and when we are not. But how do we use our intuition, or gut instinct, to help us find our way down the mountain, down to our own, personalized path to health and well-being? For me, yoga and mindfulness are the answers. It is hard to hear the messages your body wants to tell you when there is a lot of background noise, including stress, to-do lists flashing in your head, and conflicting theories. I suggest a three-step process, *the three C's,* that will allow you to listen to your body, make good decisions, and commit fully to those decisions. The three C's are:

- **Connect** to your center.
- **Commit** to what you are hearing.
- **Communicate** in an open dialogue with your body, which means being a great listener.

There are specific yoga poses and mindfulness exercises that can help you with each of the three C's. For those who are interested, please see Appendix A for a more in-depth discussion of how yoga and mindfulness can assist you in integrating all of the six mountain mantras into your life.

QUIET YOUR BODY AND KNOW
WHICH WAY YOU SHOULD GO.

Nuts about Nuts

At a recent Nurture program with fifth-grade students, I endeavored to teach them about the three macronutrients: carbohydrates, fats, and protein. It was a Friday afternoon, and the kids were losing focus. I was on the spot to have a lesson that was memorable and engaging, so I started running around the room.

"I'm really active! I need fast-acting fuel! Give me carbohydrates!" Then, I pretended to reach into my pocket for a snack. "Oooh! An almond! Almonds are nuts, which have carbohydrates."

Then I started to pretend to lift weights. I was squatting down and pulling up with my imaginary weights. As I groaned and grunted, the kids started to really pay attention. And laugh at me.

"Phew! Now that I'm done with that, I need to rebuild my muscles! I need protein!"

So I pretended to reach into my pocket again. "Oooh! A cashew! Cashews are nuts, which have protein."

Then I rubbed my tummy. "I'm still hungry. What macronutrient besides protein really helps me feel satisfied?" I pretended to reach into my pocket again. "Oooh! A macadamia. Macadamias are nuts, which have healthy fat. Healthy fat makes you feel full and helps your body at the cellular level."

I went on to explain that nuts are an example of a balanced food that contains all three of the macronutrients. Then I talked about the foods that were heavier on carbohydrates (grains, fruits, and veggies), heavier on fats (olive oil, coconut oil) and heavier on proteins (meat, poultry, and fish). To keep the kids' attention, I continued to run around the room, tapping the kids to test them on macronutrients.

"Name a food that has protein!"

Steak, lentils, beans.

"Name a food that has fat!"

Olive oil, butter, cheese.

"Name a food that has carbohydrates!"

Crackers, apples, rice.

At the end of the school year, I asked the students which lesson was their favorite.

"The one where you ran around the class like a crazy lady, talking about nuts!" one student said.

Another added, "Mrs. Guylay, we love when you come to teach in our class, even though you are a bit nuts."

MAKE HEALTHY CHOICES AND FOLLOW YOUR GUT,
EVEN IF EVERYONE THINKS YOU'RE A NUT!

A Gut Choice: Commit to Wellness

I started to really enjoy tinkering with nutrition and wellness when I came up with my own personal system that was fun and made me feel good. My system is based mostly on the primal and Mediterranean eating principles combined with: a curiosity arising from *The Omnivore's Dilemma* (by Michael Pollan) about the food chain; polished with insight from *Animal, Vegetable, Miracle* (by Barbara Kingsolver); and a desire to grow at least a portion of our family's food, inspired by *What's on Your Plate* (a wonderful book and film produced by Catherine Gund). My system is also holistic in the sense that wellness isn't just about food; it's also about movement, relationships, and even spirituality.

C   Connect to something greater than yourself.

O   Other people have a right to their own opinions.

M   Manage stress.

M   Move every day.

I   In Mother Earth I trust.

T   Techniques for cooking should be simple.

M   Meals should be about friends and family.

E   Energy in, energy out.

N   Never say never.

T   Too much of a good thing can be harmful.

Here are some details about these ten components that make up my *commitment* to wellness.

1. **Connect to something greater than yourself.** It is no fun to feel alone. I don't think we are. If you are not religious, know

that you can at least connect with Mother Nature. Just the other day, Alexander's friend Axel marveled at an idea: "Can you believe there are more stars than there are grains of sand?" This child sat at our breakfast bar and showed me the face of true wonderment. Try not to get too distracted by a myopic view of the world. Stop and remember that we are part of a vast, amazing universe.

2. **Other people have a right to their own opinions.** I have learned to avoid judging when it comes to food. I try really hard not to use the word bad when talking about food or wellness habits. Arthur Agatston, author of *The South Beach Diet*, introduced me to the concept of good fats and good carbs like olive oil, fruits and veggies, and whole grains. I love talking about food as good. It can be fun to rank a food in terms of how good it is. Agatston was the first to teach me about the glycemic index (GI), a measurement of a carb's effect on blood sugar. The GI scale goes from 0 to 100; the closer to zero, the less impact the food has on your blood sugar. Good carbs are lower on the glycemic index. They are digested slowly, so you feel fuller longer, and your blood sugar and appetite don't go out of whack. Some carbs, like mashed potatoes, give you a blood sugar rush followed by a crash. Foods with a GI under 55 are considered low, between 56 and 69 intermediate, and those above 70 are considered high. Understanding the GI scale is a great way to help you choose foods that will keep your energy steady throughout the day and avoid food-induced crashes.

If you want to evaluate your own food on the GI scale, I encourage it, but keep your findings to yourself. You might know that a plate of french fries can wreak havoc on your blood sugar, appetite, and energy level, but don't offer the information unless someone asks you. A friend scarfing down a side of fries might rather not know.

3. **Manage stress.** I mentioned previously that nutrition is directly linked to 80 percent of morbidity factors. Stress is likely linked to 100 percent. The only two morbidity factors in the top 10 that I don't consider to be related to nutrition are accidents and suicide. I can easily link these to stress. I encourage you to do what you need to manage stress in your life. The importance of stress management is a primary reason why I include yoga and mindfulness practices as key components to a wellness program. See Appendix A.

4. **Move every day.** My nickname in college was Energizer Bunny, and I was known to buzz around campus nonstop. I also was a runner, especially once I began to recognize the positive effect running has on my mood.

Another huge factor that encouraged my running was my dog Mackenzie, who pretty much forced me to run with him every day or he would destroy my tiny apartment. Need an incentive to run every day? Get a herding dog! Mackenzie kept me active throughout college, graduate school, work, and even in my early baby days.

I can't emphasize enough the importance of finding some way to get moving every single day. Exercise releases endorphins, the happy chemicals, in your brain. Keep trying methods of exercise until you find something that you absolutely love—dance, yoga, martial arts, hiking, walking, playing in the snow, biking, you name it! Talk to your doctor about starting an exercise program if you don't have one in place. Start with 15 minutes a day and work up to 60 if you can. An hour a day is the amount that Michelle Obama's Lets Move! campaign asks of kids each day, so go ahead and act like a kid.

5. **In Mother Earth I trust.** Please emphasize real food in your diet. Veggies should be your best friends. I also love nuts, seeds, and healthy oils, such as olive oil. I don't completely ban grains but stick to my favorites, which include quinoa and steel-cut oats. Following Mark Sisson's *The Primal Blueprint* series, I include high-quality dairy, which I truly enjoy. Greek yogurt is a great source of protein and calcium that is also portable for snacks on the go. I get protein with every meal in the form of eggs, dairy products, poultry and fish, or plant-based sources, such as beans, seeds, nuts, and legumes. I'll eat red meat only on occasion. I try to keep refined sugar (and white flours, too) to a minimum.

If you're able, grow your own greens and herbs or buy local when available. There is nothing more satisfying than going out to your garden before dinner and cutting greens for a fresh salad. Grow or buy dark leafy greens (like chard, kale, or even the more adventurous tatsoi and mustard greens). Dark-green leafy vegetables are loaded with nutrients: folate, magnesium, trace minerals, vitamins A and K, and the kind of fiber that satisfies. If you are not used to eating dark greens, start with a mild green, such as romaine, and experiment from there.

In the Mediterranean plan, vegetables are tossed into almost everything, including soups, stews, sauces, salads, pasta, and pizza. They are often grilled and then drizzled with extra-virgin olive oil.

Support your local farmers and know from where your eggs, meat, and fish come. Take a trip to a farm with your kids and allow your experience to transform how much value you place on food. U.S. citizens spend much less on food as a percentage of income than most other countries. We have room to grow in this area.

6. **Techniques for cooking should be simple.** Simple cooking methods ensure that I eat home-cooked meals. Our family has home-cooked meals six nights a week, with one night at a restaurant (with a shared entrée, of course). I don't think that simple has to be boring. If you want to get fancy, use herbs and spices. My friend Julia (of the ant-eaten birthday cake in Mantra #1) loves to experiment and showed me the newest addition to her cookbook library, *The Flavor Bible* (by Karen Page), the last time we visited. Julia is able to make gourmet meals right out of her rice cooker and slow cooker. You, too, can learn how to use aromatic herbs and spices to enhance flavor. I love to use fresh herbs. No dish can be ruined by adding fresh oregano, rosemary, basil, or parsley.

7. **Meals should be about friends and family.** Studies show that kids that eat dinner more often with their families get into less trouble in their teen years. Try to sit down for a family dinner at least several times a week. Express gratitude for your food, and eat slowly with pleasure and respect for the food. Enjoy the company, too.

8. **Energy in, energy out.** People don't like to hear about cutting down calories and giving up foods. Messaging has to be particularly careful, so as to not create a sense of deprivation (see next point). The downside to improper messaging with kids can involve serious consequences, including eating disorders. Again, I turn to a Nurture game that uses the power of fun to teach a lesson: Energy Balance Tug-of-War. I recently played this game with some particularly smart adolescents at a local church. (Read about it in the next section.)

9. **Never say never.** Guess how I start each and every day? With a small bowl of chocolate chips! No deprivation, and this special snack gives me motivation to get out of bed. I don't drink coffee, so a small amount of chocolate is my morning pick-me-up, even before I make breakfast. In the evenings, I don't hesitate to unwind with a delicious glass of wine, toasting with Jeff as we count our blessings. I never pass up an opportunity to taste a dessert, even if I might stick to only three bites. A happy hour, dinner, or dessert toast can be yet another chance to express gratitude in your day.

10. **Too much of a good thing can be harmful.** Our bodies are hardwired to have a preference for sweet tastes. This kept our ancestors alive when they searched out berries and fruits at the end of a long winter, but in today's world of food abundance, the sweet tooth might be our downfall. The average American consumes 130 pounds of sugar per year, up from ten pounds in the 1800s and 40 pounds in the early 1980s. One third of all the carb calories consumed in this country come from added sweeteners. Of those, sugary beverages make up half. Sugar causes tooth decay, obesity, and Type 2 diabetes and can stunt growth in children. I encourage you to cut back your sugar levels, starting with anything that is liquid and has added sugar in it. Then, start to cut down in other areas. If you consume sugary soft drinks, one of my favorite campaigns was the Pour One Out campaign* led by the Center for Science in the Public Interest. Laughing with this video might be a start to your motivation to cut down on sugar. I am always motivated by a little bit of humor, as you might already know.

COMMITMENT IS A 10-LETTER WORD, BETTER THAN "DIET"—MUCH PREFERRED.

---

 * To see the winning video from this contest, please visit www.healthysolutionsofsv.com/drink-beverages/

Energy Balance Tug-of-War

"Hey everyone, who likes to play tug-of-war?" You could see the excitement of the kids when I made this announcement.

"Awesome. I'm so relieved," one of the Nurture students said to me. "Our camp counselor said that it was time for some stupid nutrition and health lesson. We get to do this instead?"

"Yes!" I said with a smile, knowing that we were going to do both. Separately, I made a mental note to track down the counselor later.

"Let's get organized. Everyone is going to be assigned to either Team Food or Team Activity."

"Great! I'll be Team Food captain," a tall girl volunteered.

"Perfect. Now assign everyone on your team to be a specific food." I heard people shout out things like sandwich, fruit plate, granola bar, trail mix, and so on.

"I want to be Team Activity captain!" said a strong-looking boy.

"Sounds great. You assign everyone on your team to a specific activity." I heard him working with his teammates to define activities such as soccer, swimming, walking the dog, gymnastics, and more.

I handed each of my team captains an end of the tug-of-war rope.

"Okay, you can add two foods to your side." Turning to the other captain, I said, "You can add two activities." The tug-of-war commenced.

We kept adding foods and activities with equal balance, until we had about 15 kids on each side, pulling and pulling. The rope went back and forth a bit, but it was pretty steady. Then, I thought it was time to make a statement.

"Okay, you activities," I said, pointing to about half the kids on one side, "you are now foods!" They ran over to the other side of the rope.

With an unequal distribution of power, the food side took over with such force that they all flew backwards into a mud puddle. I thought the kids would be mad at me for getting them covered in dirt, but I have never seen such fun and laughter, as these kids were thrilled to get dirty.

"I guess we overate," said the group in the mud puddle, laughing.

It was time to drive the lesson home. "Tell me what you think this game tells you about wellness," I said.

One of the captains said, "To be healthy, we must balance the energy we put in our bodies—food—with what we burn through activities."

The other team captain added, "I guess weight gain happens when we put more food in than we need for activity. To build a healthy body, it is important to consume a balanced diet and engage in activities and exercise in a balanced way."

USE PLAY TO TEACH A FACT.
TUG-OF-WAR IS NOT ABSTRACT.

Commitment in the Backcountry

I recently attended an event for one of the valley's non-profits, Wild Gift, and heard a great story about commitment. Each year, Wild Gift selects a group of young social entrepreneurs that have an idea that will help solve today's global challenges through innovation. The program takes them into the back-country of Idaho on a two-week wilderness fellowship to pro-vide the inspiration, perspective, and balance that are critical to becoming agents of change. Following this intense experi-ence, fellows are provided start-up capital and expert mentor-ship to accelerate their ideas. But they need to survive the outdoor experience first.

"I learned that your training in the backcountry can be very much applicable to being an innovator in business," said Leo Pollock, an entrepreneur from Rhode Island who is working to develop a network of environmentally sustainable commercial composting facilities that can serve his entire state.

"Going up the slopes was hard, but I just had to put one foot in front of the other. That was doable. It was when we turned around—to ski down—that I started to doubt myself and my abilities! Our guide went ahead and tested the integrity of the snow, but getting down the backcountry slope skiing through the turns on icy terrain seemed overwhelming and intimidat-ing," Pollock continued.

"As I was traversing across the slope, I knew that I'd have to turn at some point, or get too far away from the group. But the turn was the scary part. At some point, it clicked that I would just have to trust my judgment, read the conditions, commit to making the turns, and carve my path down the hill. When we reflected on our day later at camp, I realized that this idea of forcing myself to commit was the same important lesson for get-ting to the next level with my business idea."

When I caught up with Pollock just a year and a half after he first incorporated The Compost Plant, his purpose and commitment had combined to create a formidable social enterprise dedicated to *changing the face of waste*. He and his team had raised funds to invest in the equipment to start collecting food waste. They had made huge strides in improving the efficiency of the processing segment of the business and were poised to create a branded product for the third phase of his business model—selling the value-added end product of high-quality compost materials to landscapers and homeowners. He had turned commitment into success.

Pollock had also recently been invited to speak at TEDx about his role in changing the world to be a better place. (TEDx presents local talks from leaders in technology, entertainment, and design.)

"We are in the business of changing a paradigm," he said to me with excitement as he shared his success stories in recruiting major universities such as Brown to participate in repurposing food waste into a community and environmental resource. He was fueled by the purpose of knowing that waste systems need to change as our landfills run out of space. The lesson about commitment that he learned while skiing in the backcountry was the key to take his business to the next level.

PRACTICE COMMITMENT TO MOVE AHEAD.
YOU MIGHT FIND YOURSELF ON TED.

Be Your Own Avatar

"As I stood in the gates before the start of a race, I would close my eyes and center myself. Then I would open my eyes, and my eyes would be huge and glowing, just like in the movie *Avatar*. I would be a superhuman version of myself."

Langely McNeal, World Cup and X Games professional Ski Cross competitor, revealed this pre-race visualization to a sports psychologist on the U.S. Ski Team. "Weird" was the diagnosis, but McNeal was encouraged to do it if it worked.

Making absolutely sure that her training techniques were successful was of no small importance to McNeal, as she risked her life every time she hit the Ski Cross course. Ski Cross is an event where four skiers start in the gates at the same time, racing against each other to finish as they hit jumps, waves, and high-banked turns, similar to a motocross course covered with snow. The big air and tabletop jumps can mean serious injury or death, given that you are flying 150 feet above ground and landing on your skis at speeds you reach in a car on a highway.

"I bond with my skis and poles in the same way that the Na'vi warriors bond with their banshee mounts," McNeal explained to me.

I thought about the scene from *Avatar* where protagonist Jake (in his avatar form) creates a neural bond with his banshee (a flying dragon-like creature) so that both rider and animal can move with power, grace, and skill through the sky. McNeal also *locked in* before a race, but not with a banshee. She would visualize becoming one with her skis and her poles. She needed this connection with her equipment to perform at what does appear to be a superhuman level.

"The *Avatar* visualization is the way that I channel my fear. You can let fear overcome you and weaken you, or you can turn it into something that makes you strong. When I open my huge, cat-like eyes as a Na'vi before a race, I feel tingles throughout my body, and I know I can do it. The gates open, and I go!*"

ENGAGE FULLY.
SOAR LIKE A BANSHEE.

Mantra #6: Throw yourself down the mountain is a reminder that once you have everything else in place—your great attitude, your foundation, your vision, goals, and willingness to learn from your mistakes—it is time to commit. Commitment requires that you overcome your fear. You can transform your fear into excitement or even love. Hawkins' map of consciousness teaches us that fear is a low state of being and doesn't allow us to be the best version of ourselves. We must first move up through anger and pride in order to experience a breakthrough with courage. From that turning point at courage, our state of consciousness helps us manifest what we want because we are in a state of positivity. Commitment also allows us to break out of the state of indecision that can lead to our ultimate demise, as we saw with the squirrel effect. Feeling that *diet* is a four-letter word, I've offered you *commitment*

* To get a taste of the McNeal Avatar experience, watch one of her GoPro videos at: www.healthysolutionsofsv.com/avatar/

instead. My 10-step framework is holistic and encourages you to make your own commitment to your wellness and well-being. As we saw with Leo Pollock from The Compost Plant and professional skier Langely McNeal, commitment is critical in every avenue of your life, from sports to business. *Throw yourself down the mountain* is about honing your ability to commit, allowing you to soar to the next levels of success in many areas of your life.

ACTION ITEMS FROM THIS CHAPTER

FOR SUCCESS IN LIFE:

- Face and embrace your fear with the knowledge that you can transform it into courage and, ultimately, into love and success.
- Engage in activities that connect you with something bigger than yourself.
- For high stakes events, channel your fear to become a superhuman version of yourself.

FOR SUCCESS ON THE SLOPES:

- Stay forward. Throw yourself down the mountain.
- Put on your Superman cape and try something new, whether it's a new run or a pond skim.
- Remember that even the best skiers in the world face fear all the time. You are not alone. Recall the major difference between excitement and fear: excitement has breath and fear does not. Just breathe.

FOR SUCCESS IN WELLNESS:

- Recognize that nutrition advice includes a controversial, diverse set of recommendations. Don't drive yourself crazy in squirrel mode.
- Develop your own individualized approach to health and wellness, using the *three C's* of connect, commit, and communicate, and adapt it to your own needs over the course of your lifetime.
- Incorporate any or all elements of my COMMITMENT plan for wellness to suit your life.

Conclusion

Thank you for joining me on my journey down the slopes and into wellness and life success. I hope you enjoyed the stories of the four winters that our family has spent in Sun Valley, Idaho.

These adventures have meant so much more to me than just learning a sport and spending time in the mountains. They helped me to finally integrate the many different pieces of my disjointed life experiences. What did running a non-profit organization have to do with a strong core? What did being a management consultant have to do with skiing into a pond? What did being an expert on efficient cooking have to do with being a gracious wedding guest? These experiences all seemed disjointed until the mountains helped me to put them all together.

On the slopes of Sun Valley, I can often be found talking to myself, either out loud or silently inside my helmeted head. I am repeating to myself a mantra (*plant your poles, plant your poles, plant your poles*) and creating success that echoes in other areas of my life (*set your goals, set your goals, set your goals*). Through the practice of associative fluency, or looking at a series of seemingly unrelated events to recognize their pattern and connection, I arrived at the cohesive six-step plan described in this book: the six mountain mantras.

Question: Can the six mountain mantras really help to make us more successful?

I answered this question just recently while I wrote this book. Here is how the mountain mantras kept me on track during this challenging process.

Change your lens on life. This mantra helped me to set the parameters of what my attitude should be for this book project. I decided early on that I'd only write this book if I could have some fun. Remembering this guideline helped me to craft this project and decide who I wanted to work with and how. If I found myself unhappy or frustrated for too long, I knew it was time to reassess and recalibrate.

Get some good boots on. I used this mantra to remind myself to make sure to do my homework and prepare. This project involved many hours of writing and a multiple of those hours spent learning about the publishing industry itself. Publishing a book is a complex process and doesn't just end with a book in your hands. I wrote a marketing plan, learned a lot about publicity, and discovered who does what throughout the entire sales chain. Of course, for the creative process itself, I put in many necessary hours to check facts and edit and revise until I felt that I had a good boot fit. And I made sure to fuel up with a great breakfast every day, so that my brain could optimally function for the serious thinking required.

Zoom out for the best view. Thanks to this mantra, I set my vision for this book at the very start. The minute I decided to do the project, I started calling myself "the author of an upcoming book." (I wouldn't even have a book title until several months later.) This verbalization was the law of attraction at work, paving the way for the book to become a reality. I wanted to involve my friends, family, and community and to follow a grassroots approach. I also wanted to make sure that I would help other people. I did visualization exercises before I went to bed at night, feeling the sensations of helping others in leading happier and healthier lives. When I woke up in the morning, I thanked the universe in advance for the guidance I knew I was going to get. What did I need to work on that day, and how could I do my best work? How could I follow my grandma's sage advice and make sure that my book was a combination of my passion and my God-given gifts and would meet a critical need in the world? I followed my dad's advice, and I wrote my vision down. I checked in with my vision periodically to make sure that I was on track, and I noticed that the ideas and people that I needed to make this project a success just seemed to show up when I needed them. I relied on my slow cooker to ensure that I could work long days and still enjoy home-cooked meals with my husband and now tween and teenage kids.

Planting my poles was critical to staying on track. I knew it was a big vision to create a book and launch it. I wanted to get it all done in what is considered an aggressive timeline for the publishing industry—well under one year. I also thought, *how great would it be to start this book when the ski lifts closed for the 2014/15 ski season and publish it by the next season opening?* Perfect timing! So I set my sights on that time frame for the book's creation. I learned from my research (Mantra #2: Get some good boots on) that a lot of the work actually comes *after* the book is published. I wanted to have fresh energy to take care of my book after it launched. I kept in mind that life is long and that I didn't have to get everything into this first book. Perhaps I will write another in the future—maybe even a whole set. I reminded myself of the concepts of incremental progress and developed a work plan that would allow me to put everything in order. When I found myself staring at a blank page, unable to craft a cohesive thought, I went out into nature or did a yoga or mindfulness practice that helped me to quiet my overtaxed brain. I found that I was able to most successfully manifest what I needed when I balanced proactivity with receptivity.

Yes, I *embraced the yard sale* (or several of them) throughout this writing process. My failures were many and diverse, from rushing to pick the title of the book (which none of my beta readers liked) to choosing the wrong structure for the book (*Mountain Mantras* was originally written in two books). In fact, I could probably write an entire separate book on the yard sales I experienced with this project. The important point is that I learned so much from these failures, am a smarter person as a result, and have a better book that will help more people and be more enjoyable to read. Health-wise, there were times when I found myself self-medicating with a portion-distortion bowl of chocolate chips as I wallowed in the misery of my mistakes. Or I missed meals or forgot to get my rice cooker and slow cooker going for my family. I tried not to beat myself up for these transgressions but instead to learn from them and get back on track. Remembering that perfection is the enemy of getting it done was key in allowing me to push ahead on a tight time frame. It's not that I didn't expect high-quality workmanship and healthy meals for my family, it's more that I couldn't expect to wordsmith every sentence for hours-on-end while serving gourmet meals three times a day.

This book was a great experience in *throwing myself down the mountain*. Of course, I often thought:

- *What if people hate the book?*
- *What if it sells only three copies worldwide (that would be my dad, my mom, and me)?*
- *What if I get laughed out of Sun Valley?*

I had to remember to follow my own advice: It was time to simply commit. I had to let go of my fears. I had to remind myself over and over:

- *I love this town of Sun Valley and this state of Idaho. I can't wait to share it with the world.*
- *I love the mountains and skiing and all that they have taught me. I can't wait to share the mountain mantras. I know they have so much to teach and can help many others.*
- *I love feeling healthy and vibrant. I can't wait to share these lessons for wellness and life.*

I learned to listen to my gut and to transform my fear into love. The answer to the original question—Can the six mountain mantras really help to make us more successful?—for me is a profound *yes*. It is my wish that this six-step plan helps you, too. Together, we can make this world a better place.

THE SIX-STEP PLAN PROVED TO BE TRUE.
IT EMPOWERED ME TO BRING THIS BOOK TO YOU.

Afterword

No two people will take away the same benefits from this book, but I do hope that you experience many tangible improvements in your life. Please, I encourage you to be in touch with me as you continue on your own journey towards wellness and success. Tell me how this book affects you and your life!

Here are some ways to stay in touch with me:

- If you are most interested in more information about my non-profit work with Nurture, please visit www.nurture yourfamily.org and sign up for the newsletter on the right-hand sidebar at the top of page. When you sign up, you will receive a free e-cookbook of slow cooker recipes. I send out a quarterly newsletter with nutrition advice, recipes, and tips on how to implement education programs in your own community.

- If you are most interested in tips for raising healthy kids, I encourage you to visit www.healthykidsideas.com and sign up for that newsletter. When you sign up, you will receive a free e-cookbook of healthy lunchtime recipes for kids. I send out a quarterly email with kid-friendly recipes, family wellness advice, and tips for getting you and your family into the garden.

- If you are most interested in corporate wellness and staying in touch regarding my speaking engagements, please visit www.healthysolutionsofsv.com and sign up for that newsletter. When you sign up, you will receive a free e-book on corporate wellness. I send out a quarterly email with resources and ideas for corporate and group wellness programs.

Each of those websites has a contact page that will allow you to send me a personal message. I am interested in your journey as you learn your own wellness and life lessons.

Repeat the mantras on whatever slopes you find yourself. Off we go!

DON'T LET THIS BE THE END.
SHARE THIS BOOK WITH A FRIEND.

Giving Back

In the spirit of giving back, I am delighted to donate a portion of the proceeds from *Mountain Mantras* to the following worthy causes:

Fast and Female U.S.

Fast and Female International was founded in 2005 by Chandra Crawford, an Olympic gold medalist in Nordic skiing in the 2006 Olympics. Fast and Female U.S. was launched in 2007 and has been hosting inspiring camps across the country in a variety of sports, including skiing, cycling, running, and multi-sports. The organization's goal is to support, motivate, inspire, and empower girls ages 9 to 19 to stick with sports and a healthy lifestyle. Fast and Female creates "empowerment through sport" for girls by hosting fun filled, non competitive programming led by female Olympians and elite athletes as well as by delivering educational content to parents and coaches. Fast and Female hopes that, one day, all girls will have positive and empowering experiences in sports as a foundation for success in life.

www.fastandfemale.com/international/usa/

Other Designated 501(c)(3) Organizations

In addition to proceeds designated for Fast and Female U.S., I am honored to partner with a multitude of worthy organizations on a rotating basis. For a list of selected organizations, please see the Resources section (Appendix B) under Non-Profit and Other Organizations.

Integrate the Six Mountain Mantras with Yoga and Mindfulness

This book would be incomplete without a discussion of how to integrate yoga and mindfulness into a life brimming with wellness and success. The word *yoga* means union, and yoga seeks to unite movement with breath. Mindfulness is the act of being aware, without judgment, in the present moment.

Both yoga and mindfulness are based on a practice of focusing on the breath. Many of us have a bad habit of using only a fraction of our lung capacity. We breathe in a shallow way as we rush through our daily activities, without slowing down to really fill our lungs. When you inhale, work on getting your breath all the way down to your belly and all the way up to your collarbone, while expanding your ribs along your sides. When you exhale, give your body the opportunity to relax.

Every yoga pose, or *asana*, has a specific benefit to the body. The cool and crazy part about yoga is that it has the ability to tap into the deeper emotional memories that can be stored in the body without our being aware of them. The mind and body are interrelated, and we tend to hold certain unresolved emotions in different places physically. You have probably heard the saying, "What you resist persists." When you deny certain emotions or don't process them fully, they can get stuck in certain parts of the body.

The mindfulness practices in this appendix are adapted from Erica Linson, a healer who helps people improve their lives through energy medicine.

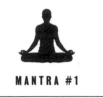

MANTRA #1

Change Your Lens on Life with Yoga and Mindfulness

In the heart and chest areas, we tend to store sadness and grief. Stretching to open these areas can liberate underlying emotions and help you let them go. Yoga is much less expensive than therapy! Try spending a few moments every day in some heart-opening poses* to maximize gratitude for life.

- **Camel.** This pose creates space in the lungs and chest and can help with respiratory ailments. Because this pose is energizing, I avoid it before bedtime.
- **Modified low lunge.** This pose opens the hips and, as a bonus, the chest. Most people lift their arms straight up into the air, but I like to put my arms into what I call goalpost or cactus positions. This helps with opening the chest and lungs.
- **Supported bridge.** Yoga should also be about relaxing into the pose and letting go. So for you type-A folks, more restorative

* To view pictures of these heart-opening poses, please visit www.healthysolutionsofsv.com/heart-opening-yoga-poses/

poses, such as the supported bridge, will likely be the most difficult for you.

EXPERIENCE LOVE AND LESS STRIFE.
HEART-OPENING POSES CHANGE YOUR VIEW ON LIFE.

Loving-kindness meditation is a great mindfulness practice to open your heart as you change your lens on life. Focus on your *heart space*. Notice what you notice, then, starting at your core, go through this outward progression of good wishes.

Starting with "I" as the object, say these words:

> *May [object] be happy and safe.*
> *May [object] be healthy and strong.*
> *May [object] be peaceful no matter what is happening.*
> *May [object] be free from suffering.*

Move outward. Make the next object your family.

Continue to move outward. The object can be your entire community of colleagues or your neighborhood, for example.

Take a moment to include a person who is giving you trouble. Yes, maybe even an "enemy" or just a really tough personality in your life. That person becomes the object of your good juju. This one is tough, I know.

Continue to move outward. The object can become your state or nation. Ultimately, you want the object to be all living creatures, planet Earth, or infinite space.

Now, how's your heart space? Notice what you notice.

This is a basic structure that you can modify.

LOVE YOURSELF AND EXPAND OUT.
A CHANGE IN THE WORLD YOU'LL BRING ABOUT.

MANTRA #2

Get Some Good Boots on with Yoga and Mindfulness

Yoga and mindfulness can be great tools for strengthening your foundation. Yoga and mindfulness help to bring some energy down and away from our busy minds and into our feet. The following three poses* are my favorite for feeling rooted and grounded:

- **Mountain.** It seems simple because you are just standing there, but there is much more to this pose. You want to get your shoulders back, tighten your abdominal muscles, and spread

 * To view pictures of these foundation-strengthening poses, please visit: www.healthysolutionsofsv.com/foundation-strengthening-yoga-poses/

your weight evenly across your feet so that you feel extremely balanced.

- **Tree.** This pose is great for getting more attention directed toward your feet, especially the one that is firmly planted on the ground. Keeping your gaze steady on a distinct focal point helps your balance. Connect with your body and listen.

- **Half moon.** Everyone has a favorite pose, and half moon is mine. I love the feeling of expansion as I reach toward the Earth with one leg and extend one arm upward. This pose reminds me of the famous quote by Theodore Roosevelt: "Keep your eyes on the stars and your feet on the ground."

Mindfulness exercises can also help you feel more grounded and increase body awareness. The following exercise aims to get you out of your head space and into your body. The headspace is the realm of the *monkey mind*, the chattering to-do lists, preoccupations of the past, and worries for the future. This exercise involves two simple steps:

1. Imagine that you have a grounding cord that begins at the base of your spine, or your feet, and extends all the way to the center of the earth.

2. Keep that image of the connection to the Earth in your mind while you start to gain a deeper awareness of your physical body. Feel your body at a deep and visceral level.

With this simple exercise, you might find that your chattering monkey mind quiets a bit. That's great progress! You might want to go a little further and ask that anything you don't need, like nervous or negative energy, simply goes down the cord into the core of the planet, where it is transformed into something positive. Feel the sense of connection to the Earth and all the living creatures that inhabit it.

When you feel like you are working from a strong foundation, you are likely to make better choices in every aspect of life. You are also more likely to listen and take steps to provide your body with good maintenance to improve your health.

GROUND THROUGH BODY AND MIND.
STRENGTH AND GROWTH YOU WILL FIND.

MANTRA #3

Zoom Out for the Best View with Yoga and Mindfulness

We have already learned that yoga poses and mindfulness exercises can open your heart and ground you. Did you know they also can help you connect with a higher source of vision and creativity?

According to the ancient system of *chakras*, energy vortexes align with areas down your central vertical axis, from the top of your head to the base of your spine. One of the highest chakras is referred to as the *third eye*, the area behind the space between your eyebrows. There are a few poses* that can activate your third eye and allow you to connect upward to gain vision.

- **Standing head to knee.** Don't let the name of this pose scare you. I can't touch my head to my knee for the life of me, unless I really bend my leg. Instead, you can put a yoga block between your head and your knee to create a connection. Think about getting a little massage between your eyes while you are in this pose—I can withstand just about anything if I am getting a massage.

- **Seated head to knee.** This is a modification of the standing head to knee pose. Here, you keep your bottom on the ground. Bend your knee as much as you need to in order to make contact between your third eye and your knee. Use a yoga block, if necessary. Don't force anything in yoga!

- **Breathing exercise.** Remember the importance of the breath in yoga. Specific breathing exercises give you time to focus on inhales and exhales. While you sit, interlace your fingers above your head. As you inhale, lower your hands behind your head. When you exhale, extend your interlaced fingers back above your head. Imagine you are moving your own halo up and down to remind yourself just how divine and amazing you are.

 * To view pictures of these third eye activating poses, please visit www.healthysolutionsofsv.com/eye-activating-yoga-poses/

You can utilize a mindfulness practice as you do your yoga poses to increase your ability to tap into a higher consciousness. As you sit and breathe, extend your awareness upward. Imagine that you have a "V" (like an old-fashioned TV antenna) that extends from behind your head at the base of your skull upward to infinity. Use the TV antenna to facilitate a connection to something bigger than yourself. Ask for some help in co-creating your reality so you don't feel like you have to do everything yourself. You don't.

REMEMBER "E.T. PHONE HOME."
MINDFULLY CONNECT AS YOU SAY "OM."

MANTRA #4

Plant Your Poles with Yoga and Mindfulness

One of my favorite parts of a yoga practice is taking a moment at the start of class to set an intention. Setting your intention is where mindfulness meets yoga practice. Setting your intention is also like planting your pole when skiing. It encourages you to ask where you want the practice to take you.

Your intentions can change on a daily basis. I've found myself asking for such things as achieving a greater sense of peace and calmness, sending love to a particular individual, or finding balance.

Some yoga poses are designed to facilitate decision-making and follow-through. Some activate the gallbladder meridian: the energy channel that starts at the head and runs down the neck, across the shoulder and down the ribs, then continues along the outside of your lower body.

Here are some goal-setting yoga poses* to consider:

- **Cow-faced pose.** I like this one because cows make me smile. I don't like it because my arms can be quite stiff, and they don't touch behind my back. Your arms are supposed to look like a cow's ears, which is what gives this pose its name.
- **Triangle.** This is one of my all-time favorite poses. Try it and you'll see why.
- **Pigeon.** Very few people are indifferent to pigeon pose. You will love it or hate it—or both. I have been in some yoga classes where people were sobbing and others where they were sighing so loudly with pleasure it almost sounded indecent. The hips represent the deepest junk drawer of the emotions. Pigeon pose might force you to dump some of those contents out so that you have to deal with them. Prepare for whatever comes and just breathe.

CLEAR OUT THE EMOTIONS WE STORE.
CLEAN UP THE JUNK DRAWER.

---

 * To view pictures of these goal-setting poses, please visit www.healthysolutionsofsv.com/goal-setting-yoga-poses/

MANTRA #5

Embrace the Yard Sale with Yoga and Mindfulness

Since very few people excel at balance poses the first time they try them, I have often thought that these poses should be called *falling down* poses. When you begin, you will likely wobble and fall over repeatedly! You learn from these wobbles and falls until you eventually can stay in balance for a longer time. Finding strength from your core and playfulness in your activities are two key concepts in the practice of yoga. Developing your balance, or the ability to stay still while standing on one leg (or head in the case of a headstand or arms in the case of arm balances), actually comes from the strength of your core. The following poses* are great for achieving balance, step by step.

- **Warrior Three.** Stand on one leg and call upon the strength of your inner warrior. Think of your body as the letter T (which can stand for whatever you like: titan, test pilot, totally awesome, or too cool for school).

* To view pictures of these balance (or falling down) poses, please visit: www.healthysolutionsofsv.com/balance-yoga-poses/

- **Eagle.** Follow the rule "Under is the same as over." To get into this pose, have your right arm go under your left arm and your right leg go over your left leg. *Test question:* How does the other side work? *Answer:* Left arm under, left leg over.
- **Headstand.** Only attempt this pose if you are an experienced yogi (or gymnast) and have a great spotter.

DON'T BE AFRAID IF YOU FALL.
YOGA CREATES CHANGES BIG AND SMALL.

While falling down is a critical part of learning, I understand that no one particularly *likes* to fall. Athletes talk about how a ski crash can be more destructive mentally than physically. That negative memory can persist and hold an athlete back until he or she can break through that limiting belief.

The same is true for many of the negative feelings or memories that may hold us back in all walks of life. To get past certain mental issues, we can utilize a mindfulness exercise that will destroy and transform that mental block. The *blow up the rose* exercise is a great way to destroy blockages. This mindfulness exercise can also transform an area in your life that feels stuck or is in need of change. Here's how to do it:

1. Close your eyes and breathe deeply. Imagine a rose floating in front of your closed eyes. It can be any color, shape, or size.

2. Imagine that rose as a representation of a belief, event, or story that no longer serves you. The rose may grow or change as you associate it with that event, belief, or story that you want to transform.

3. Now, mentally blow up the rose. As it blows apart, see how that event, belief, or story disintegrates and no longer exists.

4. Repeat this exercise as many times as you like, until you feel like the belief, event, or story no longer holds any power over you.

This mindfulness exercise taps into the fundamental power of creation, destruction, and transformation. As you mentally break up the form of your rose, you allow change to occur. Blowing up the rose is an ultimate exercise in letting go. You might need to let go of certain attachments, judgments, and expectations relating to those beliefs, events, and stories that are holding you back. When I feel stuck in my life, I love to turn whatever is holding me back into a rose and then just blow it up. Boom! Flower power.

MAKE A MENTAL CHANGE.
BRING A ROSE TO THE FIRING RANGE.

MANTRA #6

Throw Yourself Down the Mountain with Yoga and Mindfulness

When I talk to individuals and groups about improving their wellness, the car-as-body and food-as-fuel metaphors always create a connection. Most people are actually pretty good about vehicle maintenance, and they certainly get the car checked out if a warning light starts to flash. If we could start by simply treating our bodies as well as we treat our cars, we might be able to take a step in the right direction when it comes to our health. To do so, we must ask ourselves if our bodies are getting the general maintenance that they need for optimal performance, and we must certainly listen to any warning signs. But how do we look for and listen to these signals, since the body doesn't have the same indicator lights as a car?

Enter *the three C's,* a practice that combines yoga and mindfulness beautifully. The three C's* are:

- *Connect* to your center. **Forearm plank.** We learned in Mantra #5 how our power comes from our core. In yoga, the

* To view pictures of the three C's, please visit: www.healthysolutionsofsv.com/yoga-poses/

area we are trying to connect with is called the uddiyana bandha, or the stomach lock. To find this area, try exhaling while you suck your stomach up and back toward your spine. My favorite pose for creating a connection with uddiyana bandha is forearm plank. It is like doing a pushup, but you remain still, and you have your forearms on the ground to support yourself instead of your hands. Your legs are extended back as in a push-up. Try holding this pose for ten seconds, building up to a minute or more. Alexander and I often have contests to see who can hold this pose longer. We call it *resting like a Jedi*. It's so much more fun than sit-ups or your typical abdominal exercises.

- *Commit* to moving forward. **Crow pose.** Now that you are connected to your core, use this power to allow you to commit to something scary. I suggest practicing crow pose if you are having trouble with that *just go for it* moment. Crow is the art of leaning forward slowly with your knees on your triceps until one foot leaves the ground and, finally, the second foot. Crow gives you the sensation of being a bird leaving the nest. Once you have committed, you are flying. What did it feel like to just go for it? Did you notice how much core strength you needed to use to get and stay in crow? Now that you know that commitment comes from a strong center, it is time to go into listening mode. Ask your body what it feels like to connect with your center and take a leap of faith.

- *Communicate* in an open dialogue with your body. **Corpse pose.** Communication really means being a great listener, and you can do this important listening as you recline in corpse pose. Often called *savasana* (a Sanskrit word), corpse pose is the ultimate way to let go. You lie on your back with your arms at your sides and just stay there. This is when we are truly human beings, allowed to *be* instead of always having to *do*. Savasana has been the hardest pose of all for me to learn. I have been lucky to have great teachers who don't let me squirm out of doing the pose correctly, which means staying in the pose until it's time to get up. One of my teachers would severely chastise any misguided soul who dared try to leave class during savasana. Before? Fine. After? Fine. But don't dare walk out during! Corpse pose is a time when the yoga practice is fully integrated into the body. For me, it is a time when I can quiet the mind, be connected to my center, and get feedback about my commitments. It is yoga and mindfulness all wrapped up into one, and it is now my favorite pose in the yoga series. All you have to do is breathe. Listen to what your body wants to tell you. As my first teacher of Chinese medicine, Irit Steiner, once taught me: "I inhale and relax my body. I exhale and smile."

YOGA AND MINDFULNESS FIND YOUR CENTER.
INTO COMMITMENT YOU CAN ENTER.

Resources

To keep some great information at your fingertips, the following resources will be updated on the Healthy Solutions of Sun Valley website: www.healthysolutionsofsv.com. You can also access these resources at www.mountainmantras.com or follow the links or QR codes below.

Books Referenced in *Mountain Mantras*

http://www.healthysolutionsofsv.com/books-referenced-mountain-mantras/

Non-Profit and Other Organizations

http://www.healthysolutionsofsv.com/nonprofit-organizations-wood river-valley/

Snowsports Organizations

http://www.healthysolutionsofsv.com/snowsports-organizations/

Health and Wellness Organizations

http://www.healthysolutionsofsv.com/health-wellness-organizations/

About the Author

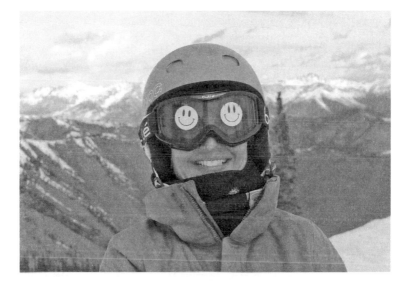

When she's not on the slopes, Kathryn Kemp Guylay is engaged in numerous other activities in her community and beyond. She is wife to husband Jeff and proud mother to Elena and Alexander. Kathryn, Jeff, Elena, and Alexander live in Ketchum, Idaho with their six pets.

As the founder and executive director of Nurture, Kathryn provides free nutrition and wellness education and services to children and families.

As a principal of Healthy Solutions of Sun Valley, Kathryn brings wellness solutions to organizations and corporations through speaking engagements and workshops.

You can hear Kathryn's voice on KDPI FM Ketchum when she hosts her own bi-weekly radio show on wellness topics. Find

out more at www.kdpifm.org and listen to her shows through
live streaming across the globe. Recordings of all Kathryn's
radio shows can be found at www.healthykidsideas.com (kids
topics) and www.healthysolutionsofsv.com (corporate wellness
topics) under the tab "Radio."

In service to her community, Kathryn acts an advisory
board member for The Hunger Coalition, the food pantry for
the Wood River Valley in Idaho. She is also a mentor at the Ketchum Innovation Center, which provides guidance and support
to small, local businesses. She is a big fan of Michelle Obama's
Let's Move! campaign and is proud to participate in several areas of the initiative. Kathryn also participates as a local ambas-
sador for the Jamie Oliver Food Revolution and the Center for
Science in the Public Interest (Food Day).

Recent awards include the Pillars of Character Award (City
of Highland Park, Illinois), the Community Health Hero (Edible
Schoolyard of Berkeley, California), and Health Hero (Public
Health Department of South Central Idaho).

Kathryn earned a BA from Emory University and an MBA
from the University of Texas at Austin. She earned her Certification in Nutritional Counseling from Trinity College in War-
saw, Indiana. Kathryn has several certifications in corporate
wellness from the Wellness Council of America (WELCOA).

Kathryn is the co-creator of the children's book *Give It a Go,
Eat a Rainbow,* in collaboration with professional food photographer, Paulette Phlipot. For more information about this book,
please see www.giveitagoeatarainbow.com.

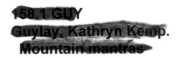